Intermittent Fasting

16/8

Delightful Recipes & Meal Plan for 3 Weeks

Lose Weight with the Revolutionary Intermittent Fasting 16/8 Method

By Carl Jackson

Disclaimer

Table of Content

Introduction

Fasting is something that has been practiced for decades and decades now, starting all the way back to the early days of civilization.

Either for religious, spiritual or health purposes, fasting has been helping individuals since the early days.

The Muslims, for example, fast during the days a holy month of Ramadan. Similar fasting events are observed in Christianity, Judaism, Buddhism and so on.

Various cultures even fast for various non-religious issues. Geneva in Switzerland, for example, holds the "Fast of Geneva", which is a nice holiday celebrated in September by people of Geneva.

Rooted in the Middle Ages, the main purpose of these fasting was to act as a sort of penitence after various wars, plague or epidemics.

Recently, however, with the advancement of modern sciences, more and more people are now aware of the amazing benefits that entail the process of fasting, and as much, more people are trying to incorporate fasting in their daily lifestyle.

They are not doing it out of spiritual faith or tradition, rather they do it because they want to reap the amazing advantages of fasting and stay healthy for days to come.

So, what is intermittent fasting then? Well, Intermittent Fasting is the process of cycling between periods of fasting and feeding windows following a number of different programs and protocols.

Since no two human beings are alike and all of them have their own weakness and strengths, multiple forms of intermittent programs are created to allow an individual to find the best one that suits their lifestyle.

At the time of writing, Intermittent Fasting stands as one of the most popular processes of both staying healthy and losing weight!

Due to its rising popularity, it has been seen that the number of online searches tailing the word "Intermittent Fasting" has increased by almost 10,000 percent since 2010 and still growing!

The main aim of this amazing booklet is to work as a complete guide that is meticulously crafted to give you all the basic concepts and knowledge that you are going to need in order to get them right into the world of intermittent fasting!

You should understand that the core focus of this book is the 16:8 protocol where you are encouraged to eat for 16 hours while keep fasting for 8 hours.

We chose this particular program because this is essentially the most accessible one of the bunch.

However, we have still covered all the basics of intermittent fasting in chapter 1 alongside some awesome information in chapter 2, 3 and 4 that will significantly help you in your journey.

All of these are followed by a sample 3 weeks meal plan designed to inspire you and create your own plans using awesome recipes provided in this book!

I hope that you will enjoy the experience with this book and it will be helpful to you.

Chapter 1

Core Intermittent Ideas

The first chapter of this book will cover all the fundamentals concepts of Intermittent Fasting and more.

We have lots of details of cover, so I will try to break everything down into smaller portions in order to make it easier for you to digest.

So, before we even dive into what "Intermittent Fasting" is, we must first understand the core fundamentals of "Fasting" first.

What if Fasting?

When people talk about fasting, the word "Starvation" often comes to mind that immediately creates a negative impression on those who are unaware. But you should understand that there is a very drastic difference between "Starving" and "Fasting.

Throughout this book, we are talking about "Fasting", keep that in mind moving forward.

So, let's clarify that first.

You should understand that the concept of fasting is different from starvation in the sense that one is done due to not having any option while the other is intentional and controlled.

People starve because they don't have anything to eat, while people fast because they choose not to eat.

People who starve often have no plan as to what they will have as their next meal or even where will it come from.

They don't intentionally starve, rather the situation makes it rather difficult for them to gain any sort of food. Scenarios such as these often are created during events times of famine or war when food becomes extremely scarce.

Starvation is forced upon an individual while fasting relies completely on how you want to consume your food.

On the other hand, Fasting is essentially voluntarily keeping yourself away from food for health, spiritual or other reasons.

During times of fasting, food is readily available for you to consume, but your self-control prevents you from consuming them.

The choice is completely up to you in this case.

This option of having a "Choice" is what ultimately helps draw a line between fasting and starving.

You should keep in mind that fasting and starving are not the same things! And no, none of those two terms are interchangeable with one another. If you have a good understanding, then you would notice that both of them completely opposite in meaning.

And on that topic, you should know that general fasting does not really have any fixed duration, rather the duration depends on what kind of fasting you are doing.

As a quick example, you can simply look at Ramadan which is the month of fasting for Muslims and learn how to get rid of bad habits.

 You will understand this concept better once we explore intermittent fasting further.

Consider the term "Breakfast", have you ever wondered why is it called "Breakfast"?

It's essentially because, after dinner, you don't generally consume anything and go to sleep, in the morning, you are breaking your fast by eating something.

Hence, breakfast.

The word itself acknowledges that fasting is far from a cruel punishment and is something that is performed on a daily basis, albeit for a short time.

And not to mention, Fasting is also considered as being an "Ancient Weight loss Secret" by many!

Got your attention now didn't I?

Well, now that the basics of Fasting are covered up, let's move forward and dive into the core topic of our book, which is "Intermittent Fasting".

What is Intermittent Fasting?

Now, let's have a look at what "Intermittent "fasting really means.

In contrast to fasting, the term Intermittent Fasting simply is a method of specifying certain periods of time when you will fast, and this fasting has to be continued regularly to achieve all benefits.

The amount of time you will fast and the period of your eating window will depend on which protocol you decide to adhere by.

While there are many different types of intermittent fasting programs, there's not really a "Best" one that will cover the needs of everyone. And that is exactly why the different programs exist.

They all work to a certain degree for different individuals, you have to find the one that will work best for you.

You should know that the effectiveness of protocols might vary from person to person. So you might need to do a little experiment in order to find the perfect one for you.

You should know that the length of fasts might be anywhere from 12 hours or more and fasting can be followed for one week, two week or even a few months. It will depend on your program and your desired weight target.

However, in general, shorter fasts generally are followed more frequently, daily if needed, while the longer ones such as the ones that last for 24-36 hours are usually done 2-3 days a week.

Unlike most other programs, Intermittent fasting won't force a fixed diet regime upon you, rather it will allow you to eat whatever healthy food you want to eat, following your desired eating pattern.

To summarize, even more, the intermittent fasting program will ask you to intake 0 calories meals and food for a set period of time, which will be followed by low-calorie foods of your choosing during your "Eating" periods.

As mentioned earlier, there are actually multiple types of intermittent fasting program, each of which are designed for a specific type of person.

You will find brief discussions of all the major protocols in this chapter, but to give you an overview, below is a list of the main protocols that you should know about.

- Spontaneous Meal Skipping
- Warrior Diet
- Alternate Day Fasting
- 5:2 Protocol
- 16/2 Method

What are the different types of Intermittent Fasting?
With the core concept out of the way, the next thing that I believe you should know about is the different types of intermittent fasting protocols that are available to you.

Yes, you heard that right!

There's much more to intermittent fasting that to just stopping to eat and eating again when the right time comes.

Due to the demands and physiological conditions of different human beings, scientists and nutritionists have crafted out a number of different types of intermittent fasting protocols.

Each of these different types of protocols is designed to cater to a specific type of audience.

While there are lots of different programs, below are some of the core ones that you should know about.

Spontaneous Meal Skip: This protocol does not come packed with a specific fasting period and rather works on giving you the freedom to choose your very own time frame.

Which means if one fine morning you don't feel hungry, you can simply skip breakfast on that morning and fast till dinner and have a healthy meal to top it off. Alternatively, you may also skip lunch and dinner and have breakfast!

The whole point of the protocol is to give you the freedom to make your fasting routine.

Alternatively, you may also opt to skip lunch and dinner and breakfast altogether. The whole point of this plan is to allow you to make the most perfect and beneficial plan for you.

The Warrior Diet: This particular program was created by one expert known as "Ori Hofmekler" and according to him, the best way of fasting is to expose yourself to as many vegetables and fruits as possible.

Keeping that in mind, Ori moved forward with his particular plan that further inspired people to eat very little portions of vegetables and fruits throughout the whole day and making sure to end the day with a nice and hearty meal.

After dinner, you are required to completely fast for 4 hours at least and continue the cycle once again.

Alternate Day Method: This particular method will require you to simply fast for any particular day and then choose to skip fasting the next day. To make things clearer, if you fast the whole day today, you are allowed to skip fasting for the next day.

The thing about this that you should know is that there are actually a number of different variations of this particular protocol. So, make sure to do your research and choose the one that suits you. Regardless, the main aim of all the protocols is to keep your calories under 500.

Also, this form is very similar to the well-known "Eat-Stop-Eat" protocol, which is also discussed below.

Eat-Stop-Eat Protocol: This particular form of Intermittent Fasting will ask you to fast for about 24 hours for twice or once a week and it is strictly prohibited for you to eat anything during that particular period. And do the opposite during the other days.

To make things clearer, you can have your first meal at 7 AM on one day, then eat nothing until 7 AM of the coming day.

This particular program has been made famous by fitness Brad Pilon.

The 5:2 Diet: This particular program asks you to eat healthy food for 5 days a week while making sure that you keep your calorie intake under 500-600 calories per day.

As for the fasting part, you are to simply fast for the next 2 days.

This particular form of fasting is extremely popular in America.

And just in case you are still not clear about the protocol, what you essentially have to do is eat on all days except for Tuesday and Thursday. On the alternate days, what you must do is simply eat normally, making sure that you keep your calorie under a limit of 500 and break up those calories into small-sized meals.

The 16/8 Method: The 16/8 method is the core method that I will be explaining throughout the chapter since this is often believed as to be the most accessible and effective one.

This protocol is very simple as it will just require you to have a fasting window of 14-16 hours daily and have a feeding window of 8-10 hours.

It makes things easier for you, you can start off your day by having a meal at 8 AM in the morning, after which you may count 10 hours and keep feeding appropriately. Once you are done with that, you are to fast for the next 16 hours.

This cycle will keep on going. And just for the record, during your fasting window, you are allowed to drink "Zero Calorie" beverages like coffee or water.

Benefits of Intermittent Fasting?

Intermittent Fasting is one of that programs that comes packed with a bucket load of amazing benefits.

Fasting plays a very important and crucial role in multiple cultures and religious activities, and for good reason!

The advantages that one can enjoy from an intermittent program is fascinating.

Below are eight amazing benefits that you will enjoy and that are even proven by science!

Blood Sugar Levels: Multiple thorough research have shown that regular fasting significantly helps to improve the level of sugar in your blood, which in turn helps to numb down the possibility of your body suffering from diabetes in the future.

Alternatively, another study showed that fasting greatly increases your sensitivity to insulin.

Helps fight inflammation: Inflammation is a serious issue amongst a lot of people. What happens during chronic inflammation the cells of your body starts to attack itself, which leads to various illness such as heart disease, arthritis, and even cancer.

This is a serious issue and I have dedicated a whole chapter for discussing inflammation, so don't worry!

Enhance heart health: If you have a look at the larger picture, heart diseases are considered as being one of the leading cause of deaths all around the world, in fact almost 31.5% deaths globally take place due to heart diseases.

One small study has seen that intermittent fasting helps to lower down the levels of bad cholesterol by almost 25% and triglycerides in the blood by almost 32%.

Boosts brain power and strengthens mind: Even though research in this field is limited, there are multiple studies that have shown that fasting can have a very positive effect on your cranial health.

Another study involving mice following intermittent fasting for almost 11 months showed significant improvements in brain structure and function.

Since it helps in lowering down inflammation, it greatly helps to deal with neurodegenerative diseases as well.

Helps to lose weight: I have already talked about this extensively, but since you are limiting your calorie intake during an Intermittent program, you are significantly improving your chances of losing weight.

But that's not the only factor here though, but there are also many more factors to consider here that I have discussed in coming sections of the chapter.

Improves longevity: Multiple animal studies have shown that with Intermittent fasting, they were seen to have improved longevity and lifespan.

In a recent study with rats, it was seen that rats who fasted every alternate day lived for 83% longer than rats who didn't fast.

Other reports with different animals show similar results.

Helps in the prevention of cancer: Studies with various animals and test-tube studies have seen that fasting might actually help to a greater degree when it comes to preventing and treating cancer.

One study with rat showed that alternate-day fasting helped him to completely block the formation of a cancerous tumor.

Another similar study using a test tube showed that introducing cancerous cells to fasting had a similar positive effect to chemo when it came to delaying the grown of cancerous cells.

There's much more than the ones that are mentioned above! The above ones were given just to give an idea of what you are getting into.

What is 16:8 Intermittent Fasting?

I have already briefly discussed a little bit about the 16:8 Intermittent Fasting program, let me discuss it further now.

SO, the 16:8 or 16/8 intermittent protocol will ask you to limit the consumption of your food and any kind of beverage that you increase your calorie count for about 8 hours and fast 16 hours of the remaining day.

You are actually allowed to keep following the 16:8 protocol for as many days as you require until you are able to reach the body fitness and health level that you were planning for.

In recent years, the 16/8 protocol has gained lots of popularity and is especially one of the prime protocols that newcomers tend to follow when wanting to burn more fat and lose weight.

Why should you choose 16:8 Fasting?

The 16/8 Intermittent Fasting protocol is particularly attractive for beginner fasters and for good reason.

While most other programs tend to impose upon you a very restrictive set of dietary rules, the 16/8 program doesn't do any of that!

In fact, this is a very simple and easy to follow diet program and will allow you to bring in awesome results with minimal effort.

Due to the versatility and flexibility of the protocol, it is rather easy for any individual to seamlessly squeeze this program into their daily lifestyle.

In addition to helping you to lose weight, the 16/8 program also will help you to improve your cranial functionality, improve your sugar levels and increase your overall longevity.

So, if this is your first time trying fast, the 16/8 is possibly the perfect and best option for you!

And even if you are fasting veteran, the 16/8 will also help you to wind down a bit from your more hardcore fasting programs while still being able to enjoy the benefits of fasting.

Guidelines for Intermittent 16:8

Now that the basics of the 16/8 protocol are covered, let me walk you through how you can actually start following the program.

I have already laid down the ground rules of the program, so let's dig deep.

So, the first step for you to do is to choose your fasting window.

We already know that you need to fast for 8 hours right? So let's talk about that.

Many people opt to eat between the noontime and 8 PM at night, this allows individuals to cut a good chunk of fasting time and after the last meal, they can just go to sleep.

Afterward, you can simply have a balanced and healthy dinner and lunch in order to maintain your daily calorie intake.

On the other hand, some people tend to eat between 9 AM and 5 PM, which will give you enough time to have a healthy breakfast at around 9 AM, have a fine lunch at noon, a light dinner or snack at around 4 PM and finally start your fasting for 8 hours.

But the above mentioned two were just simple examples, you are allowed to choose your very own plan as you need.

You should keep in mind though that during your "Eating" window, you must prevent yourself from overeating, otherwise nothing will work out.

The meals and snacks should be spaced out properly in order to help your body adjust with your blood sugar levels and appetite.

Also, if you want to further enhance the effectiveness of this program, you should try to stick to unprocessed "whole" food and healthy beverages.

A good way to deal with this is to balance out your meals by having meals that include ingredients such as:

- Poultry, fish, meat, eggs, nuts, seeds, etc. for protein
- Coconut oil, avocados, olive oil as your healthy fat
- Rice, oats, barley, buckwheat, quinoa as your healthy fats
- Tomatoes, leafy greens, cucumber, broccoli, cauliflower, etc. as your veggies
- Orange, apple, bananas, berries, peaches, pears as healthy fruits

During your fasting periods, you are allowed to go for calorie-free simple beverages such as water or even unsweetened coffee or tea and they will help you stay hydrated and control your appetite.

And as mentioned earlier, if you eat more and more junk food, then all the positive effects of the 16/8 program will be negated and it might ultimately do more harm to your health than good.

To summarize, this particular protocol of Intermittent Fasting is really easy to get into and is a hassle-free way of experiencing how fasting works if you haven't already.

Plus, it gives enough feeding time so that you don't feel incredibly weak and allows your body to slowly adjust itself to the physiological and cellular changes that are accompanied by the protocol and fasting itself.

What to eat while fasting and what not to eat

While there are no specific food guidelines as to how you should make up the "Eating" portions of the day, we recommend that you try to stay away from processed food as much as possible and stick to natural alternatives.

Healthy Fats: It is really good for you to consume healthy fats when staying in a clean eating diet. Go for the following

- Olive oil
- Extra Virgin Olive Oil
- Organic Unsalted Butter
- Coconut Oil
- Organic Ghee
- Sunflower Oil
- Avocado

Flours and Grains: Always make sure that you are using 100% whole grain flours that have no additives or preservatives.

- Bread
- Pasta
- Tortillas
- Rice
- Flours
- Soba Noodles
- Cornmeal
- Bread Crumbs

Dairy: Always go for full-fat organic and grass-fed dairy products.

- Plain yogurt
- Buttermilk
- Greek Yogurt
- Sour Cream
- Cream Cheese
- Cottage Cheese
- Milk
- Cheese

Nondairy/Protein Alternative: For protein alternatives, it is good to go for unsweetened plain almond, soy sauce, coconut milk, or even rice.

- Organic Tofu
- Organic Tempeh

Seafood: Sustainable shellfish and fish are the best choices when considering seafood.

Produce: Organic products such as vegetables and fruits are always great for a clean diet.

Meats: When going for meat, it is essential that you go for hormone and antibiotic-free organic meats.

- Poultry
- All-natural bacon
- Uncured deli meats such as ham
- Lean red meats

Salts and Herb: Salts and herbs are self-explanatory. Use them in reasonable amounts.

- Herbs
- Kosher salt or sea salt

Nuts: Nuts as seeds are allowed in a clean diet, so use them liberally

- Unsalted nuts and seeds
- Organic unsalted seed butter/ nut butter

Sweeteners: It is essential that you keep your sugar intake to an as low level as possible, but if your sweet tooth is tingling too much! Then simply go for the following CE approved sweeteners.

- Raw honey
- Date sugar
- Pure maple syrup
- Stevia
- Organic Evaporated cane juice
- Dark chocolate
- Pure vanilla extract
- Unsweetened shredded coconut

Juices: Always go for 100% pure juices!

- Lemon juice (100%)
- 100% fruit juice
- Cold-pressed or homemade 100% vegetable and fruit juices

Thickeners: Some thickeners are allowed in a clean diet such as

- Arrowroot

- Tapioca Starch
- Potato Starch

Canned and Jarred Produce: For canned goods such as tomatoes or beans, only go for the ones that are BPA free.

Condiments: One thing to note while purchasing condiments is to look for the labels. Make sure that they contain no additives, preservatives or sugar. Alternatively, if possible then try to make your own.

- Hot Sauce
- Dijon Mustard
- Reduced Sodium Soy Sauce
- Vinegar

Some additional ingredients: Some more that you should know about:

- Dried berries that are unsweetened
- Liquid smoke naturally crafted
- The chicken broth that is low in sodium
- Agar
- Tomato paste (unsalted)

How to identify processed food

The quick pointers below will help you to a clearer idea of how you can identify processed foods.

- ✓ Foods that contain any kind of preservatives such as salt, flavor or sugar in order to extend their shelf life are processed food. This includes beverages as well as breakfast cereals.
- ✓ Any kind of food that has its natural form altered should be considered as processed food. For example, bread with their bran and germ removed are to be considered as processed food.
- ✓ Foods that contain one or more artificially created components are considered as processed food.

How should you calculate your calorie intake?

This is something that you should pay very close attention to as having a proper calorie intake/burn rate is crucial to how much weight you will lose in the long run.

You may have noticed while browsing through various food labels that the given values are specified to be "Percent of daily values". Now, you might be curious as to know what does that exactly mean.

Well, it means that those particular nutritional values are presented and calculated considering a scenario where an average person eats 2000 calories in one day. But this is not made in stones as the physiology and requirements of every single human being varies from one to the next, and your daily intake might be greater than 2000 calories.

Other factors that come into consideration are height, age, weight, gender and your level of daily physical activity.

Now, before you set up your weight loss target, it is important that you know how should actually calculate your daily calorie intake.

While calculating your daily calorie intake, there are certain factors that you are to consider and keep in mind, such as:

- Thermic effect of food
- Physical activity
- Basal activity

And as for the actual procedure, we need to talk about something known as "BMR".

Just in case you don't know, the Basal Metabolic Rate is the minimum level of calorie required by your body to keep it healthy in a resting state.

This particular value amounts to almost 60-70% of the calories that you burn each day. Keep in mind that generally speaking, men have a much higher BMR than women.

While there are many ways of calculating this, the most prominent method of calculating the basal metabolic rate is through the usage of the "Harris Benedict" method, which is illustrated below:

Adult male: 66 + (6.3 x body weight in lbs.) + (12.9 x height in inches) - (6.8 x age in years) = BMR

Adult female: 655 + (4.3 x weight in lbs.) + (4.7 x height in inches) - (4.7 x age in years) = BMR

Once you have figured out your BMR, the next step would you to calculate your total calorie requirements.

To do that, just simply follow the given steps based on your level of activity

- If you have almost no physical activity, then calculating your calorie intake is as simple as = BMR value x 1.2
- If you have the tendency to do light exercise and/or workout around 1-3 days per week, then your calorie calculation would be = BMR value x 1.375
- If you tend to do moderate levels of workout, around 3-5 days per week, then your calorie intake would be = BMR x 1.55

- If you have the tendency to do high levels of exercise, mainly around 6-7 days per week, then your calorie intake would be calculated by = BMR x 1.55
- And lastly, if you do very hard physical exercise/ sports activity, then your calorie intake should be calculated using= BMR x 1.9

Let me give you an example to makes clearer.

So, let's consider that you are sedentary and have low levels of physical activity.

You calculate and find out that your BMR is 1745.

So, multiplying it by 1.2, you would get 2094, which is the total amount of calorie that you need daily in order to maintain the current weight level of yours.

Calorie for losing weight

Now that the basic concepts of calorie intake are cleared up, the next step for you is to understand how you can actually start to lose weight while with that knowledge.

So, the first thing that you must understand is that there are approximately 3500 calories in a pound of your stored body fat. So, if you want to lose body fat, what you have to essentially do is burn 3500 calories either through dieting or physical exercise, or using both of them combined.

If you are able to create a calorie gap of 7000, then you will be able to burn 2 pounds in a week. The amount of stress that your body is able to take will ultimately depend on your own will power and stress levels.

The calorie deficit can be brought upon by either eating less or eating low-calorie food/having more physical activity.

The most preferred way is to have a combination of a healthy diet and a good amount of physical activity in order to get the best out it.

If you want to lose your weight, the general guideline that you should follow is to lower your calorie intake by at least 500, but making sure that you don't cross 1000 at it might hamper your normal activities.

On the other hand, if you want to lose just a small amount, then 1000 calories might be too much, so go for lower deficit targets.

As recommended by the American College of Sports Medicine or ACSM, your calorie intake should never drop below 1200 per day if you are a female and 1800 if you are a female.

Next, we will talk about how Intermittent Fasting affects the hormones of your body. But before that, let me clear up what "Hormones" actually are.

What is Hormone?

To keep things simple, Hormones are a type of a molecule that is generated in the "Endocrine Glands."

These molecules tend to influence significantly various functions of our body, including sexual functions, metabolism, development process, and growth.

A correct balance of these hormones is hugely crucial to the physical and emotional well-being of human beings. Hormones have also been studied to influence your mood significantly!

Asides from adequately maintaining the functionalities of your body, Hormones also act as messengers that travel through the bloodstreams and allows the body's various mechanism and organs to communicate with each other.

There are a bunch of different hormones in your body, and they have been classified into various types a well.

Understanding how Intermittent Fasting affects hormones

Incidentally, fats aren't the only component of your body that will be affected by your intermittent fasting program.

Asides from fat, there are several other things that will change at a cellular level, and all of these changes will be governed by changes in hormones in your body.

For example, as you carry on with your diet program, your body will alter your hormone levels so that the body is more accessible.

And at the same time, your cells also start to repair broken or worn-out cells and alter the expressions of your genes.

More details of the hormones of your body are provided in chapter 2, but for now, let's have a look at the core ones that will be affected by your fasting routine.

- Insulin: As you fast more and more, the level of your body's insulin will drop drastically. This will ultimately make your fat more accessible.
- Cellular repair: Once you fast, your body will start to repair itself through a process known as "Autophagy" where your cells will start to digest and discard the old and broken proteins that are built up inside the cell.
- Human Growth Hormone: Fasting will increase the amount of human growth hormone by almost 5 folds, which will significantly improve the rate at which your body will lose fat or gain muscle.
- Gene expression: While fasting, Gene expression changes will also take place that will help to increase the strength of your immune system and increase longevity.

Why intermittent fasting is an awesome weight loss tool

So, if you are going into the Intermittent Game, it's pretty much sure that asides from staying healthy, you must possibly want to lose weight as well right?

As you can already tell, the key to losing weight here is by increasing lowering down your calorie intake.

When you are fasting during intermittent fasting, you are automatically cutting down you're your calorie intake by consuming lower amounts of food.

Asides from that, fasting will also facilitate the hormones such as the growth hormone and lower down insulin that will ultimately make your body fat much more accessible and easy to burn. This will happen due to the increased release of another hormone named norepinephrine that encourages the burning of fat.

Because of the changes in your hormone levels, fasting might even increase your overall metabolic rate by an amount of 14% at most!

So, long story short?

Lowering down your food intake, changes in hormones caused by intermittent fasting will altogether significantly improve your chances of losing weight.

And these are not just words of mouth! A recent 2014 review study shows that intermittent fasting significantly improves your chances of losing weight over 3 to 24 weeks by close to 8% when compared to other common weight loss programs.

Another study shows that people who follow the intermittent fasting program loses almost 4-7% of their belly fat. These body fats have the tendency to significantly cause problems to the organs in the thoracic region, so it's a huge plus.

Further study also shows that intermittent fasting allows your body to reduce the amount of muscle loss, allowing your body to stay fit and rigid for a prolonged period of time.

Regardless of the benefits though, you should keep in mind that the effectiveness of intermittent fasting will ultimately depend on how well you are able to restrict your food intake.

If you fast for the whole day and eat huge amounts of food in the next, then the end result won't be satisfactory at all.

So, try to keep your daily calorie intake under 500, eat healthier food, workout, and fast in balance for best results.

Intermittent fasting is an awesome tool indeed that accelerates the process of fat burning, but its effectiveness will depend on how well you are able to control yourself in the long run.

Some precautions to keep in mind

If you think about it on a broader perspective, you would notice that unlike most diets, the only side effect of an intermittent dietary program is that during the early days of your diet, you might feel very hungry.

However, the thing to keep in mind is that hunger often has the tendency to bring general weakness along with it, which in turn might make you feel lethargic to some extent.

You don't have to worry too much about this though as eventually, the feeling of lethargy goes away as your body adjusts itself to the new form of diet.

However, you should keep in mind that if you have any of the following medical condition, you should consult with your physician before embarking on the fasting journey.

- If you have diabetes
- If you are suffering from any kind of blood sugar regulation problem
- If you have low blood pressure
- If you are on regular medication
- If you are underweight
- If you have a history of eating disorders
- If you are female who is trying conceiving
- If you are female with a history of amenorrhea
- If you are a pregnant or nursing mother

Now that everything is pretty much cleared up, below you will find a simple meal plan that is designed to inspire you to make up your own plan.

Now since we are specifically dealing with the 16:8 plan here, the meal plan below is designed in such a manner.

3 weeks 16:8 meal plan

So the way the plan is designed is that, for every day, you are fasting from 11 PM to 7 AM, while during the other time periods, you are having 3 meals, dividing them between intervals of 4-5 hours with minimal snacks in between.

Week 1

Week 1	11 PM – 7 AM	Meal 1	Meal 2	Meal 3
Day 1 (Sunday)	Fasting	Eggs In A Hole	Collard Greens	Tuna Croquettes
Day 2 (Monday)	Fasting	Delicious Pumpkin Pie Oatmeal	Cauliflower Cake	Grilled Lime Shrimp
Day 3 (Tuesday)	Fasting	Hearty Pancakes	Broccoli And Cauliflower	Blackened Chicken
Day 4 (Wednesday)	Fasting	Eggs In A Hole	Collard Greens	Tuna Croquettes
Day 5 (Thursday)	Fasting	Delicious Pumpkin Pie Oatmeal	Cauliflower Cake	Grilled Lime Shrimp
Day 6 (Friday)	Fasting	Hearty Pancakes	Broccoli And Cauliflower	Blackened Chicken
Day 7 (Saturday)	Fasting	Tomato And Egg Scramble	Collard Greens	Western Pork Chops

Week 2

Week 2	11 PM – 7 AM	Meal 1	Meal 2	Meal 3
Day 1 (Sunday)	Fasting	Hearty Pancakes	Mouthwatering Calamari	Spiced Up Kale Chips
Day 2 (Monday)	Fasting	Pineapple Oatmeal	Broccoli And Cauliflower	Asparagus Tart
Day 3 (Tuesday)	Fasting	Egg Muffins	Zucchini BBQ	Paprika Lamb Chops
Day 4 (Wednesday)	Fasting	Hearty Pancakes	Mouthwatering Calamari	Spiced Up Kale Chips
Day 5 (Thursday)	Fasting	Pineapple Oatmeal	Broccoli And Cauliflower	Asparagus Tart
Day 6 (Friday)	Fasting	Egg Muffins	Zucchini BBQ	Paprika Lamb Chops
Day 7 (Saturday)	Fasting	Egg Muffins	Zucchini BBQ	Spicy Meatballs

Week 3

Week 2	11 PM – 7 AM	Meal 1	Meal 2	Meal 3
Day 1 (Sunday)	Fasting	Roasted Broccoli	Collard Greens	Spiced Up Kale Chips
Day 2 (Monday)	Fasting	Pineapple Oatmeal	Leeks Platter	Coconut And Cauliflower
Day 3 (Tuesday)	Fasting	Egg Muffins	Chicken Garlic Platter	Garlic And Kale
Day 4 (Wednesday)	Fasting	Roasted Broccoli	Collard Greens	Spiced Up Kale Chips
Day 5 (Thursday)	Fasting	Pineapple Oatmeal	Leeks Platter	Coconut And Cauliflower
Day 6 (Friday)	Fasting	Egg Muffins	Chicken Garlic Platter	Garlic And Kale
Day 7 (Saturday)	Fasting	Egg Muffins	Zucchini BBQ	Spicy Meatballs

Chapter 2

Additional Information for Your Journey

Key nutrients to know about

Fasting will put a lot of stress on your body and since you will be missing out on food for a long time, you will need to ensure that you are having a well-balanced diet in order to make sure that your body is healthy.

Below is the core nutrition that you should focus on.

- **Protein:** These are also known as the building blocks of our body since they help to generate and heal a different kind of tissues in our body. They promote growth and development.
- **Fat:** While people often look at Fat in a negative way, these are also essential as they act as a backup reservoir of energy for the body.
- **Carbohydrates:** Carbohydrates are the primary source of energy in our body. They range from simple to complex and are often very easily converted to energy.
- **Water:** Water helps to maintain the optimum level of homeostasis in our body and is responsible for allowing the body to easily transport nutrients all around.
- **Minerals:** Aside from the main nutrients, there are essential minerals that are needed to trace amounts in order to maintain a healthy body. For example, Potassium helps to maintain optimum cell fluid level, calcium strengthens the bones and so on.
- **Vitamins:** Similar to minerals, Vitamins are also needed in trace amounts to ensure that the body is functioning properly. Lack of certain vitamins often leads to a severe health problem. For example, Vitamin C is responsible for collagen synthesis, which helps to maintain the blood structure, on the other hand, Vitamin D helps to ensure that the body's calcium homeostasis level is maintained correctly.

Once you are cleared up on the nutrition, have a look below to know more about some awesome healthy food alternative to common daily ingredients.

Healthy alternatives to common ingredients

Since our book is actually about Ketogenic Desserts, you can already tell that sweeteners are going to be at the center of every recipe.

It is very crucial that you know about the Low-Carb "Keto-Friendly" natural sweeteners that you are allowed to use while on a Keto Diet. These sweeteners will help you elevate the flavor profile of your dessert while not bulking it up with excessive carbohydrates or sugar.

You should understand that there are many different types of sugar substitute, and they generally come under various brand names.

That being said, the most common ones that you should know about are as follows:

Stevia: Stevia or "Stevia Extract" to be precise is the extract of the stevia plant that occurs naturally in the wild. It is a zero-calorie sweetener and so is perfect for the diet. You can find them in either liquid form or powder form. For most recipes, using the liquid form is suitable; however, it is advisable that you keep the liquid version nearby as well as they are perfect for liquid-based recipes. While purchasing Stevia, make sure to buy the one that does not have any added ingredients, as some brands tend to pack up their products with various artificial ingredients.

Erythritol: Contrary to Stevia, Erythritol is a naturally occurring substance that is commonly found in various cheese and fruits. Similar to Stevia though, Erythritol is also a calorie-free sweetener that is perfect for the diet. However, one property unique to Erythritol is that it has a kind of "Glaze" like appearance. This makes it perfect to be used as icings or coatings. One important thing that you should keep in mind while using Erythritol is the fact that the flavor that this produces is 1:1 to sugar. That means that 1 tablespoon of Erythritol will give you the same flavor as using 1 tablespoon sugar.

Swerve: Swerve is a powdered artificial sweetener that is available in both superfine and granular textures. This is equally sweet as sugar, so you should use it accordingly.

Xylitol: Xylitol is a type of substance that is categorized as sugar alcohol. Just in case you don't know, Sugar Alcohols are a hybrid mixture of sugar molecules and alcohol molecules. Their unique structure gives them the property that allows them to stimulate the sweet receptors on your tongue. These substances are naturally found in many fruits and vegetables and are usually found in crystal forms in the market.

Splenda: Splenda is simply sucralose. It changes the texture of many baked goods and are almost 600 times sweeter than sugar but doesn't come packed with as many calories.

Agave Syrup: Agave Syrup is about 1.4 to 1. 6 times sweeter than your normal sugar and is generally used as an alternative to sugar or honey in recipes. It has a high sweetness factor because, at its heart, it is composed of about 70-90% fructose.

However, keep in mind that this is not an ideal sweetener, and if you decided to use it, you should use it in very small amounts.

Monk Fruit Powder: Monk Fruit, also known as the "Longevity Fruit" is a fruit that is native to China and Northern Thailand. It is almost 300 times sweeter than sugar and has been used in Chinese medicine to treat obesity and diabetes. This product is pretty much similar to Stevia regarding taste but eliminates the bitter aftertaste that is associated with most Stevia based products.

After sweeteners, the next ingredient that you should know about are the flours that you should use while making your desserts.

Regular wheat flour is packed with a load of carbohydrates, so it is obviously off the table to Keto Diet, but there are some pretty good alternatives out there.

The good ones to know about are:

Konjac Flour: Konjac Flour is a type of flour that is obtained from tubers of various species of Amorphophallus. It is a type of soluble dietary fiber that has a structure very similar to pectin. Konjac Flour mainly consists of glucomannan, which is a compound composed of glucose and mannose. It is excellent as a gelling agent, film former, thickener, emulsifier, and stabilizer.

Flax Meal: These are also known as "Ground Flax" or "Linseed" and are extremely nutritious. These are amazing sources of Vitamin B1, Copper and Omega 3. What makes Flaxseed good regarding baking is that you can use Flax Meal to replace the flour and also eggs in recipes. Most Flax Meal products that you will find in markets come in vacuum-sealed bags and boast the only 1g of net carb per serving.

Coconut Flour: Coconut Flour is an extremely Keto-Friendly flour. However, you should be wary of your quantities. However, you should also know that coconut flour is extremely absorbent, which means that just a small amount of coconut flour is perfectly fine to achieve the effects of using a large amount of wheat flour. Coconut Flour is finely ground, dried coconut flesh that is milled into a fine powder and is an excellent flour alternative for Keto baking.

Almond Flour: Almond Flour is prepared from blanched or unbleached almonds. Blanched almond flour has a smoother texture than the ones created from unbleached flour, which makes it popular for low-carb baking. Almond flour has a higher amount of fiber and protein as opposed to wheat flour and can have a much less drastic effect on your blood sugar levels. These are also packed with magnesium, potassium and other essential nutrients that are crucial to a Keto Diet.

Another ingredient that is very crucial to Keto Baking and various desserts is Milk. As you may already know, animal milk is prohibited in the Ketogenic Diet, primarily because it is packed with a very high amount of carbohydrates. The Carb to fat ratio of Milk is 5:1, which is very high! Good alternatives to animal-based milk are:

- Almond Milk

- Hemp Milk

- Macadamia Milk

- Cashew Milk

- Coconut Milk

- Hazelnut Milk

Asides from the above-mentioned flours, milk replacements, and sweeteners, the following are some of the other ingredients that you should add to your shopping list to prepare your pantry for the journey.

To make things easier, I have divided the commonly used ingredients into different categories.

Protein: When considering protein, try to buy organic whole eggs. Asides from that, good sources of Keto-Friendly protein that you might need for desserts include:

- Cashew butter

- Almond butter

- Macadamia nut butter

- Soft Goat's Cheese

- Hard Swiss Cheese

- Cheddar Cheese

- Hard Parmesan Cheese

- Soft Cheese

Chocolates: When buying chocolate for your dessert recipes, you must be aware of buying dark chocolates that are 90% or darker as they tend to have fewer carbs.

Fruits: Most large fruits are prohibited in the Keto Diet due to their large sugar content. However, you have the option always to balance your portions when using the fruits. Good Keto-friendly fruits to consider are:

- Avocado

- Raspberries

- Strawberries

- Blueberries

Fats and Oils: while on a Keto Diet, it is essential that you know the difference between good and bad fat, as these are going to be your primary source of energy. In short, unsaturated fats are the ones that you should avoid. Saturated and monosaturated fats are beneficial to the body and help to lessen inflammation. Good sources that you should consider buying include:

- Coconut Oil
- Ghee
- Avocado Oil
- Macadamia Nut Oil

Nuts and Seeds: Nuts and seeds are really good options to munch on while on a Ketogenic Diet as you can eat them with no preparation. These are also amazing ingredient to be used in Desserts. However, keep in mind that some nuts and seeds tend to be high on carbohydrates, therefore keep your portions in check. Good ones include:

- Pumpkin Seeds
- Cashew Nuts
- Pistachios
- Almond
- Sesame Seeds
- Brazil Nuts
- Macadamia Nuts
- Flaxseeds

Vegetables: Vegetables growing above the ground are mostly low in carbohydrates and are allowed in a Ketogenic Diet. Some of these vegetables are good to be used in desserts as well. Just make sure to avoid starchy veggies such as potatoes!

- Lettuce
- Celery
- Romaine Lettuce
- Kale
- Cucumber
- Spinach
- Cauliflower
- Broccoli

- Cabbage
- Brussels Sprouts

Good salt alternatives to know about

Salts are another breed of ingredient that we commonly use every day! However, we also know that consuming too much salt can often lead to high blood pressure levels, hypertension, and various other problems.

Sunflower Seeds

Sunflower seeds are fantastic salt alternatives, and they give a sweet nutty and slightly sweet flavor. You may use the seeds raw or roasted.

Fresh Squeezed Lemon

Lemon is believed to a be nice hybrid between citron and bitter orange. These are packed with Vitamin C, which helps to neutralize damaging free radicals from the system.

Onion Powder

For those of you who don't know, Onion powder is a dehydrated and ground spice that is made out of onion bulb. The powder is mostly used for seasoning in many spices! Keep in mind that onion powder and onion salt are two different things.

We are using onion powder here. They sport a nice mix of sweet, spice and bit an earthy flavor.

Black Pepper Powder

The black pepper powder is also a salt alternative that is native to India. You may use them by grinding whole peppercorns!

Cinnamon

Cinnamon is a very popular and savory spice that comes from the inner bark of trees. Two varieties of cinnamon include Ceylon and Chinese, and they sport a sharp, warm and sweet flavor.

Flavored Vinegar

Fruit-infused vinegar or flavored vinegar as we call in our book are mixtures of vinegar that are combined with fruits to give a sweet flavor. These are excellent ingredients to add a bit of flavor to meals without salt. Experimentation might be required to find the perfect fruit blend for you.

As for the process of making the vinegar:

- Wash your fruits and slice them well

- Place ½ a cup of your fruit in a mason jar
- Top them up with white wine vinegar (or balsamic vinegar)
- Allow them to sit for 2 weeks or so
- Strain and use as needed

Various Hormones and their Functions

Previously in the first chapter, I already discussed the different types of hormones that will be affected by intermittent fasting.

Some core ones that you should know about are listed below:

- Oxytocin
- Testosterone
- Adrenaline
- Estrogens
- Vasopressin
- Melatonin
- Insulin
- Prolactin
- Thyroxin
- Growth Hormone

Let me break down the functions of the type for you.

Growth Hormone

Just to let you know, Growth hormones are extremely essential for the proper functioning of your endocrine; And these are secreted by your pituitary gland that is finely situated at the bottom base of your brain.

It also helps to maintain your body fat levels and keep them at optimal levels while protecting your body against cholesterol.

It also helps to improve blood circulation.

Thyroxin

These are also secreted by your thyroid gland and are produced in your body's pituitary gland. This type of hormone is generally known as "T4" and plays a significant role in maintaining bodily metabolism.

This also plays a vital role in maintaining your psychological health.

Prolactin

These are secreted in the adenohypophysis under the brain and are mainly responsible for the secretion and production of milk from the mammary glands.

Insulin

These are produced by Beta Cells in the pancreas and are responsible for keeping your blood glucose level in check. They help to "Open" up the cells so that they can absorb glucose from the bloodstream.

Melatonin

Melatonin is secreted by Pineal Gland and is primarily known as the "Sleeping Hormone." This is because it helps to regulate your sleep cycles (amongst other functions) and acts as a biological clock for our body.

It also helps to strengthen our immune systems.

Oxytocin

Oxytocin is primarily known as the "Birth Hormone," This particular hormone has a multitude of functions. Amongst others, it helps to properly maintain and regulate your CNS by letting your body adapt to various different social behaviors. The part of your brain known as "Hypothalamus" is responsible for these.

This particular hormone also helps to relax your muscles and generate breast milk while you are lactating.

Testosterone

The Testosterone is the sex hormone that helps in the development of multiple secondary sexual characteristics such as pubic hair, sperm, and sex organ development.

Asides from that, these hormones are also responsible to elevate your sexual mood to the next level and maintain optimal sperm production.

Just in case you are wondering, these are produced by adrenal glands situated in ovaries in case of women and testicles in case of men.

Adrenaline

Known as the "Fight or Flight" hormone and maintains the "Survival" instincts of our body.

If your body senses any danger, it triggers a "Fight or Flight" response, which affects the body-altering blood pressure, pupil sized and heart rate, to maintain the body for the situation that it is facing.

Estrogens Vasopressin

Just like Testosterone, Estrogens are sex hormones mainly found in the female body. They also have very similar functions as Testosterone and helps to develop secondary female sexual properties such as breast development.

It is also responsible for the development of the female menstrual cycle.

Estrogen levels in a female gradually decline throughout the life cycle of women, which leads to menopause.

They also provide cardiovascular protection and stimulate the production of pigmentation and collagen in the skin.

The Harm of Misbalancing Hormone

As you already know, Intermittent Fasting is designed to encourage you to fast for a very long length of time! This particular act might end up putting your body through some negative effects, especially this is your first time!

And one of the major issues that you might face during this period is an imbalance in your hormones.

To help you understand why this is important, have a look below:

Growth

If you experience a deficit of Growth hormone, it will cause fatigue and weaken your muscle. The distribution of the body will also be in jeopardy, and your cholesterol levels will increase.

You should know that deficiency in "Growth Hormone" can very well lead to dwarfism.

Specific mood disorders linked to this hormone include social isolation, loss of self-control, anxiety, etc.

Oxytocin

Deficiency in this particular hormone might often lead to depression and multiple types of anxiety issues. Not to mention, autism is also suspected to be related to low oxytocin levels.

Testosterone

Low levels of testosterone are related to various diseases such as diabetes, obesity, depression, osteoporosis, erectile dysfunction and so on.

Alternatively, a high level of testosterone in women may lead to androgyne disorder, acne, excessive body hair, aggression, and abnormal menstrual cycle.

Adrenaline

Excess levels of adrenaline in our body can lead to harmful situations such as chronic stress and various anxiety disorders such as panic attacks or generalized anxiety.

It is also believed to have links with cardiovascular conditions, insomnia, obesity, and weakening of the immune system.

Estrogens

Estrogens imbalance leads to irritability, depression and frequent uncontrollable mood swings.

Deficiencies of estrogens production can lead to serious problems such as ovarian, uterine and breast cancer.

It also has links to memory loss and osteoporosis.

On the other hand, excess estrogen also leads to the development of tumors and amenorrhea.

Vasopressin

Constant deficiency of Vasopressin leads to diabetes insipidus and sodium deficiency.

Melatonin

Low levels of Melatonin have been linked with sleeping disorders, various inflammatory symptoms, and aging.

Insulin

Imbalance in insulin can often result in the development of hypertension, diabetes, and cysts in ovaries.

Prolactin

Excess secretion of Prolactin leads to menopause and insufficiency of Prolactin is linked to Sheehan's Syndrome. Just in case you don't know about it, in Sheehan's Syndrome, the woman's pituitary gland might be destroyed after giving birth to a child.

In the case of men though, excess of prolactin can result in various hormonal disorders and larger abnormally sized breasts.

It may also lead to erectile dysfunction.

Thyroxin

The most common dysfunctions related to thyroxin deficits include:

Hypothyroidism: In this situation, the body fails to produce the desired amount of thyroxin, which might lead to weight gain, depression, etc.

Hyperthyroidism: In this situation, the body overproduces due to hyperactivity of the gland that results in insomnia, tremors, anxiety and so on.

That pretty much covers the basics of your hormones and the issues that might arise if you face any sort of deficiency.

Next, we shall talk about obesity. But before you understand obesity, it is crucial that you have a good understanding of BMI and the core concepts of body weight.

The core concept of Body Weight

Everybody these days is always talking about losing their weight and turning into the next hot diva or mister universe! But have you ever wondered what they are referring to? Scientifically speaking course! Well, the answer is pretty simple. By the term "Weight" they are referring to the amount of mass on our body. Which is the bulk amount that comes from all the water, body fat, bones and muscle of our body which altogether comprises our skeletal and humanoid infrastructure?

When someone is called "Obese", in the simplest of sense it is usually being said that they have an excess of body fat around their exterior or interior which has exceeded the safe levels and is now harming the health of the body.

Professionals such as Doctors or Nurses often follow something which is called the BMI or Body Mass Index.

In simpleton language, the BMI is a method of measurement which is done by comparing both the height and weight of a person to come out with a rough idea of the person's physique. The formula below is used to calculate the BMI of a person.

$$\text{Body Mass Index} = \frac{\text{Weight (in kg)}}{\text{Height}^2 \text{ (in m)}}$$

Once the Index has been obtained, a similar chart to the one below is observed to assess the results.

The standards of the chart above have been set by the World Health Organization who proclaim that a BMI of anywhere between 25-30 usually results in a person being overweight while 30+ would deem him/her obese.

Sadly, though, at the time of writing, the level of people suffering from obesity and a high body fat percentage was an all-time high. In fact, in 2014 it was estimated that almost 600 million adults were suffering from obesity while 42 million of the total obese population were children under five! Thank you for excellent fast foods!

So, the next and most crucial question in everyone's mind is that, does a Ketogenic Diet or a High-Fat Low-Carb Diet help to water down the level of fat?

From the chart above, you will easily be able to assess if you are under the category of being underweight, normal, overweight or even being obese.

What is Obesity?

In strictly general terms, Obesity is a physical condition which a person faces when he/she has gathered an unusual level of fat in their body.

When your fat levels get at levels such as these, the body slowly starts to go through various bad effects that significantly hamper the condition of your heart and health.

At the moment of writing, nearly 2 in every 3 adults in America were found to suffer from Obesity, which pretty rounds it up to 68.8% if the population being obese.

The measurement of how much obese a person can come from a calculation made to figure out the BMI (Body Mass Index) of a person. It is generally considered that if the bodyweight of a person is 20% greater than the estimated value, then he/she is obese.

Current situation of America

That being said, it is really sad to say that the current condition of Americans is not pleasant. It is actually nothing short of an epidemic!

In fact, it has recently just been seen that almost 2 individuals our every 3 adult individual in America fall are checked as being overweight! On the hand, 1 individual out of every 3 is obese while 1 out of every 20 is obese.

The problem is not limited to only adults too! As $1/3^{rd}$ of the total population of children falling between the ages of 6-19 are largely considered to be either overweight or obese.

To bring things down to statistics, almost 60% of Americans are overweight while 35% are recorded as obese.

Why should you care?

As mentioned earlier, the easiest way to check if you are obese or not is to calculate your BMI.

• 25-29.9 means you are overweight
• 30+ means you are obese
• 40+ means you are extremely overweight

Aside from completely destroying your self-confidence and make you feel depressed all the time, going obese has some very serious implications for your health.

- It will increase your cholesterol levels
- It will make you prone to suffering from diabetes
- It will increase your blood pressure
- You will be more prone to health diseases
- You will be prone to suffering from a stroke
- You might start to suffer episodes of momentary breathlessness during sleep
- Your bones will weaken and you will suffer from Osteoarthritis
- The possibility of gallbladder stone formation will increase
- It will make it difficult for you to properly control your cognitive functions
- If will increase the risk of cancer
- It will cause many troubles to patients of Asthma

So, it of utmost importance that you don't let yourself go into the world of foods. Without proper control of your dietary intake, you might soon be facing severe consequences in the long run.

What contributes to Obesity?

A key factor in reducing weight through Intermittent Fasting is to have a good understanding of what "Obesity" actually is and what are the contributing factors at play.

If you have a better understanding of what makes you fat, you will easily be able to cut them down and improve your chances of losing more weight.

When talking about obesity, we often related to food.

But that's not really where everything ends as there are more factors that largely contribute to obesity alongside a heavy diet. Some of the more essential ones which you should know about are:

- **A general lack of energy balance:** This is true. If the energy input and out of your life is not balanced properly, then you will start gaining weight. The equation goes something like this:
  - Same energy input and Same energy output = no weight change
  - More energy input and less output = weight increases
  - More energy output and less energy input = Weight decreases

  And where is the energy coming from? Excessive amounts of food and drinks of course!

- **A result of your gene:** Yes, to a large extent, obesity is a condition that might be heavily influenced by genes passed on from your parents or ancestor. The offspring are obese parents are more like to suffer from obesity in the future, when compared to those of leaner parents.

- **The volley of junk food:** The days of using natural food ingredients is almost gone! Every now and then you are faced with a product that is excessively deliciously, yet is completely made using chemicals and artificial produces. These "Hyperpalatable" junk foods take a huge toll on our body.

- **Food Addiction:** Linking from the "Hyperpalatable" junk foods. Some people often get addicted to these foods, since they are both delicious and cheap. This is in fact certified as a very complex medical issue to deal with and from a biological standpoint, is very tough to overcome.

- **Lack of Sleep:** This might come as a surprise to our "Night Owl" readers. But this is, in fact, something which should be considered. Recent studies performed at the University of Warwick has shown that people who tend to sleep less are prone to suffer from obesity much more in the future.

- **Medications:** Sleeplessness in combination with a high functioning lifestyle often influences people to go for various pharmaceutical drugs such as antidepressants and antipsychotics. These drugs have the tendency to alter the working mechanism of the brain by forcing it to store more fat rather than burning it.

- **Pregnancy:** This is a natural process of life. As you get older the muscles of your body will tend to give away and become lost. If you don't maintain a properly healthy and active lifestyle, then weight gain is inevitable. For women, however, it should be kept in mind that after menopause (and pregnancy) women usually gain about 5 pounds. If this is not toned down in the future, it might lead to obesity.

These are just some of the important but crucial issues which you should keep in mind.

Preparing yourself for the journey ahead

The following two steps should help you better realize your problems and help you create a mindset that will inspire you for the days to come and help you create a solid mental foundation for the journey.

Controlling your subconscious: The human mind is a very mysterious object and even to these days, the working pattern of the brain is yet to be fully discovered. But that doesn't necessarily mean that our understanding of the mind is feeble.

The mind, in general, has two different forms of consciousness. The sub-consciousness and the super-consciousness. The super consciousness is what we are experiencing spontaneously, the sub-consciousness, on the other hand, is a layer of energy that is hidden beneath.

For people who are suffering from Obesity, this inner layer usually tends to project highly negative energy which always ejaculates a negative reason for every positive thought that might come to mind.

It is essential that as a first step, the negative energy of this sub-conscious is brought under control. A mindset should be established that won't look for reasons to "Not" do a work. Instead, it will focus on how it will be able to fully help the individual to become more determined in performing the given task. Which, in our case is dieting.

Accepting that you have a problem: Once you have transformed your mind into considering that it is now ready to undertake any task. The next thing which you should do is accept that you have a problem.

Believe it or not, obesity denial is actually a thing! And it can work largely as a negative catalyst in this case. Believe it or not, about 70% of the American population deny to believe that they are obese and take no steps towards it! This has to be changed.

Awesome tips to prevent overweight

Aside from the above-mentioned techniques, there are very simple and easy to follow tips that will greatly help you prevent excessive weight gain.

- Always make sure that you are drinking plenty of water

- Always keep vegetables in your diet
- Try to get rid of high calorie and tempting foods
- Keep yourself busy to avoid food temptation
- Don't eat between meals
- Don't skip your meals

To further accelerate your weight loss process, there are certain diets that might also interest you.

This book will be focusing on the Clean Eating diet, but asides from that there are also the following ones, which are highly effective and efficient.

Awesome tips for fasting

Now, let's talk about some amazing tips that will greatly help you during your fasting hours.

- Before beginning your fasting hours, make sure to drink as much water as possible as it will help you to stay hydrated throughout the fasting hours.

- Stay busy: It'll keep your mind off food. Try fasting on a busy workday. You may be too busy to remember to be hungry.

- You may drink 0 calorie coffee as it acts as a mild anti-suppressant and will help you to keep your appetite in check. Black Tea and home-made broths are good options.

- Hunger comes in waves; it is not constant. When it hits, slowly drink a glass of water or a hot cup of coffee. Often by the time you've finished, your hunger will have passed.

- Most people will try to discourage you simply because they don't understand the benefits of fasting. A close-knit support group of people who are also fasting is often beneficial, but telling everybody you know is not a good idea.

- Fasting is a slow and steady process, so make sure to give yourself enough time before you expect results. Just make sure to don't get discouraged.

- During your non-fasting hours, make sure to go for nutritious meals and if possible, stick to diets that are low in sugar and refined carbohydrates and are high in healthy fats.

- This is the most important tip I can offer, and it has the greatest impact on whether you stick to your fasting regimen. Do not change your life to fit your fasting schedule—change your fasting schedule to fit your life. Don't limit yourself socially because you're fasting. There will be times during which it's impossible to fast, such as vacations, holidays, and weddings. Do not try to force fasting into these celebrations. These occasions are times to relax and enjoy. Afterward, you can simply increase your fasting to compensate. Or just resume your regular fasting schedule. Adjust your fasting schedule to what makes sense for your lifestyle.

- After your fasting session, try to prevent yourself from binge eating, during your eating window as it won't help you at all. Eat normally and pretend that fasting never happened.

Chapter 3

Detoxifying your body

You may look at this 3rd chapter as being a bonus one, but the contents of this chapter will still help you to a greater degree.

So the core concept here that I want to clarify here is that, before you start intermittent fasting and losing your weight, there are certain steps that you can take in order to increase the chances of your weight loss.

Today's community of edibles has been largely marred by produces that are scratched with harmful chemicals and dangerous toxins.

Cleansing or Priming your body is the first step to essentially detoxify your bloodstream in order to give you a much more healthy internal mechanism. This will both help to strengthen your immune system as well as beautify you to a certain extent.

Let's start by talking about some of the foods that you should try to avoid first hand. Cleaning is the first step to leaning!

So, what does Detox mean exactly?

What is a Detox Diet?

Generally speaking, detoxification is a process that our body performs on a regular basis to keep the body free from harmful chemicals known as "toxins".

Now these toxins are generally divided into two different categories

- **Endotoxins:** These are the molecules that are made inside the body as byproducts of the body's regular metabolism.
- **Exotoxins:** These are the molecules that are introduced to the body by an external means. They can come through eating, breathing, drinking or through skin absorption.

Examples of Endotoxins include lactic acid, urea and microbe waste products. Alternatively, examples of Exotoxins include pesticides, pollutants, tobacco chemicals, mercury in seafood, car exhaust lead and air pollution, etc.

Since all of these toxins are possess the ability to greatly hamper the normal working condition of the body and potentially damage human health, the body tends to regularly get rid of these through various means such as through defecation, urination, respiration, and sweat.

How detoxification works actually varies vastly from one person to the next.

This fact is truer mainly because the whole detoxification procedure depends vastly on what kind of lifestyle you are following and the form of your diet, amongst some other factors.

Safe to say, that all of these different factors greatly vary from one person to the next, which ultimately influences the effectiveness of the detoxification process.

You should know though that increased levels of toxins might cause certain problems to your body. Below are some of the core ones that you might face once your body fails to eliminate the accumulated toxins.

- You might get blurred up vision
- You might experience loss of memory
- You might experience CNS disorders
- You might gain more weight
- You might face inflammation
- Colon cancer risk might increase

Detoxification actually helps to a great extent to prevent things such as these.

Detox programs often require people to get rid of processed foods or a specific type of foods such as dairy, eggs, gluten, red meat or peanuts and so on.

Junk Food

Junk foods are basically those edibles that are extremely high in calories, fat or sugar very little to no nutritional values. High protein food such as meat that is prepared with saturated fat may also be called Junk food. These are often believed to be extremely unhealthy and they tend to pose long term threat to the health of a human. Such foods include

- Sugar/ Refined food such as Twinkies, Donuts
- Products of Fats and Hydrogenated Oil such as Cookies, Chips, Candy Bars, Bologna
- Foods containing excessive salt which includes Pretzels or much-canned produce
- Fast Food such as Pizza, Burger, Fried Chicken, Sausages
- Snacks including Hot Dogs, French Fries, Pop Corns, Pancakes
- Carbonated Beverages such as Pepsi or Coca Cola

We are telling you here to completely relinquish them from your life. But maintain a balance a lower down your exposure to them.

Fermented Food

The case of fermented foods is a peculiar one, to say the least. On one hand people these days are mindlessly boasting the positive benefits heralded upon us by Fermented food.

These simple claims were simply based keeping in mind the fact that easily fermented food were the ones that helped to keep our predecessors hearty and healthy. Basically, what they did was just eat natural food!

It should be kept in mind that our ancestors were not exposed to the polluted chemicals and harmful toxins as we today. Whenever that fermented food was consumed by them, they only filled up the necessary natural requirements of their body which kept them healthy. The fact that our body has now become habituated towards artificial produces is the very reason it is not capable of enduring the raw contents of nature.

However, in our case, things are not necessarily the same. There is a limit up to which the body is able to endure natural produces, after which a negative effect start to take place. In most cases, an excess of fermented food leads to bloating, bacteria build-up and of course, gas builds up.

Some of the fermented foods include:

- Yeasted Bread
- Vinegar
- Mushrooms and Truffles
- Nuts and Seeds
- Melons
- Beer/Wine
- Fermented Soy
- Old Cheese

A Group of Inflammatory Food

Commonly, the word inflammatory is looked upon as being "aching of joints". However, things are a little bit different here when it comes to food. Inflammatory foods are basically those produces that have the tendency to turn on specific "disease" genes that are capable of turning into something serious such as type 2 diabetes and also obesity. These include

- Food Allergens
- Red Meats
- Dairy Products
- Yolks
- Nori Seaweed
- Tilapia
- Catfish
- Duck

- Yellow Tail
- Processed Sugar and Starch

How to Detoxify then?

With that said, just keeping that harmful food away won't completely detoxify you! The following steps are going to go to a large extent in order to help you to completely detoxify your body.

- **Water down excess sugar intake:** This is very important and you should start off your journey by doing this. This can be looked at as a seasonal detox that will help you increase your overall health and metabolism.
- **Drink more and more water:** Water, the essence of life. You should always make sure to, therefore, start off your day by drinking a good amount of water. In fact, starting off your day with a tall glass of water just a tint of lemon helps to completely rehydrate the
- **Don't remain static:** Even though this might be tough for some individuals considering the amount of time they have. But it is highly recommended to make a schedule to do some daily exercise. It not only helps to get lean, but it also aids blood circulation and improves the lymphatic system. It is also said that it helps to improve digestion, lubricate joints and increase the overall strength of the body.
- **Go for the Tea:** Especially Green Tea is possible. These are awesome herbal solutions to detoxify your body and keep you hydrated at the same time.
- **Try to go for Organic food:** Try to keep your food palate full of fruits and vegetables of various colors. These are full of macronutrients which your body will require and will take you to great distances in the long run.
- **Try to avoid environmental pollution:** Easier said than done. Given the level of pollution and allergens all around us. However, it is highly advised that you always flush your nasal pathway using a Neti Pot which will greatly help you to eliminate the side effects of air pollutants and help you to breathe normally.
- **Go for Sauna every now and then:** Sweating as much as possible is a great way to detoxify your body. And what better way to sweat while meditating rather than going for a Sauna bath!? Every now and then you should take some time out just for yourself and get for a Sauna bath. You will leave the room completely refreshed.
- **Scrub the dirt off:** Spiders tend to shed their skin whenever possible to rejuvenate themselves. Humans can do the same, albeit in a less scary way! You should always take some time to brush your skin and undergo oil massages to fully exfoliate the toxins from your outer skin and refresh yourself.

With these steps in mind, you will be able to greatly increase the effectiveness of your program.

Chapter 4

Regarding Inflammation and you should fast to protect you from it

I have already mentioned that Inflammation is a really big topic and it's a great deal that fasting actually helps to deal with it.

I believe that having a good understanding of Inflammation

What is Inflammation?

In the strictest terms, Inflammation is the process of the body through which the body's white cells and their accompanying substances tries to protect the body from any kind of infection due to foreign body contamination such as virus or bacteria.

It all sounds good, right?

However, in certain diseases such as Arthritis, the defense mechanism seems to malfunction and the immune system tends to trigger off the inflammatory response even when there are no foreign invaders inside the body.

Diseases that tend to do these are largely known as "Auto-Immune" diseases and instead of protecting the body, the body's own auto-immune system starts to harm itself and damage the tissues

What Causes Inflammation?

Various factors come into play when considering the reasons as to "What" causes inflammation in a human being. More often than not, a vast majority of the reasons tend to directly link to poor Lifestyle choices, however, it should be noted that aging is a big factor here as well.

Some of the most crucial causes to know about include:

Diet

If we make a comparison, we would soon see that most of the causes of Inflammation are related to diet, so we are keeping this on the top of the list.

Harmful substances such as refined fats, animal products, and refined carbohydrates tend to do a lot of damage in the long run.

It should be noted though that carbohydrates don't directly contribute to inflammation, refined foods with higher concentration and fats are found to be naturally dense with an inflammation-causing substance that affects that gut and increases inflammation.

The types of fat that are consumed by an individual also plays a greater role here. Back in the early days when everything was simple, people used to stay on a diet that was very well balanced on both Omega 3 and Omega 6 fats. However, modern diets tend to have a very high concentration of Omega -6 fat as opposed to the Omega 3 fat, this increase the possibility of suffering from inflammation by 10-20%!

It's very important for the body to have a good supply of Omega-3 fatty acids because of the Omega 6 and Omega 3, both compete for the same COX enzymes, which are needed to build large fatty molecules.

COX-2 enzyme, in particular, is essential for making inflammatory prostaglandins.

Too much of Omega-6 fatty acids will result in the domination of this enzyme and the body won't be able to utilize this enzyme anymore in conjunction with Omega-3 fats to reduce inflammation.

Nowadays fats are even chemically modified and this plays a greater role to inflammation as well. They are made to be more inexpensive, which results in the production of highly inflammatory products.

Aging

The natural process of aging contributes to Inflammation as well. As we age, few of our cells tend to regenerate and most of them start to die, leaving behind waste materials that tend to trigger inflammation.

Obesity and Inactivity

Excessive inactivity can and will often lead to obesity, which itself is a major cause of inflammation.

Adipose tissue, the layer of fat that is found right under our skin is actually responsible for much more than just keeping it warm.

It is a metabolically active layer that causes the body to change the body chemistry and is also affected by the body's other systems.

The fat layer contains a large number of white blood cells and a remarkable quantity of fat (obviously).

However, the cell count is actually linked together. Meaning, the more fat there are, the greater the number of white cells will be present.

These cells often tend to release pro-inflammatory substances that gradually contribute to the rise of inflammatory effects.

Sleep Deprivation

Researchers have shown that a lack of sleep is directly linked to the formation of certain infection-fighting white blood cells such as T-Cells. Depriving ourselves of sleep will cause the number of T-Cells to decrease, which will, in turn, increase the number of inflammation-promoting cytokines.

Stress

Cortisol is a hormone that is produced by adrenal glands and is used to manage the body's response to stress.

It helps to stimulate the burst of energy and suppresses the action of the pro-inflammatory substance.

This also helps to reduce stress by counteracting the effects of pro-inflammatory eicosanoids. However, If you stress too much, the amount of cortisol might increase to a dramatic level that will cause your immune cells to lose the sensitivity to this hormone and trigger inflammation.

Sun Exposure

This might seem a little bit surprising, but excessive exposure to sunlight can often result in an individual suffering from inflammation.

Too much sunburn or exposure encourages the formation of free radicals under the skin surface. Just to let you know, free radicals are unstable molecules that tend to destroy injury-fighting cells and lowers down the number of white blood cells present in the body.

As you may already have guessed, this lowers down the strength of the body's immune system and leads to inflammatory attacks.

Smoking

Exposure to various toxins such as cigarette smoke plays a great role in Inflammation. Either second hand or firsthand, inhaled tobacco tends to extensively cripple the body's capacity to fight diseases by suppressing the production of white blood cells.

So, it's best to avoid smoking as much as possible.

The Science of Inflammation

Now that you have a little idea of just how much "Severe" of a problem Inflammation is, let's have a look at how Inflammation works and what happens to your body during Inflammation.

Let's go back to the beginning once again, whenever your body needs to respond to an injury, it tends to mobilize an army of specialized cells to fend of the invading organism and toxins.

These cells prepare pathways for fighter cells to attack and completely engulf the attackers.

Once that has happened, another group of cells tends to signal the body and let it know that the fighter cells have accomplished their task and the body is allowed to stop the production of preparatory and fighter cells.

These results a sort of cleanup that clears up the leftover fighter cells from the battlefield repairs any caused damaged.

Simply put, there are two steps to this response:

- Pro-Inflammatory
- Anti-Inflammatory

Each cell that is involved in the pro stage builds upon the work of the previous cells and helps to make the immune reaction stronger for an upcoming attack.

During the pro period, symptoms such as redness, swelling itching are common.

The Anti-Inflammatory is the reverse of Pro-Inflammatory and it works to lower down the effects of inflammation.

A number of various substance that is used to block inflammation are made from essential fatty acids, which the body isn't able to produce on its own.

These acids must be obtained through supplements or foods.

Two essential ones are Omega -3 and Omega -6.

Omega 6 ten to increase inflammation while Omega 3 helps to reduce it.

It should be noted that what I wrote above is an over-simplified version of the whole mechanism and there's a lot more to that.

There are various substances and play a deeper role in the whole infrastructure that allows the body to control its inflammatory mechanism.

Some of the crucial ones are:

- **Histamine:** White blood cells near a site of injury tend to release a substance known as histamine. They increase the permeability of blood vessels around the wound that signals fighter cells and other substances to regulate immune response and come to the sight of injury. Histamine also causes redness and swelling around the affected region and causes a runny nose, rash, itchy eyes, etc.
- **Cytokines:** These are proteins that are activated by pro-inflammatory eicosanoids to signal fighter cells to gather at the injury site. They are responsible for diverting energy from the body to catalyze the healing process. Release of this substance tends to cause tiredness and decrease appetite.

- **C-Reactive Protein:** Cytokines alongside other pro-inflammatory eicosanoids are closely involved in the activation of a substance known as C-Reactive Protein. This particular organic compound produced by the liver responds to messages that are sent out by a white blood cell. The C-Reactive proteins tend to bind the site of injury and act as a sort of surveillance unit that helps to identify the invading bodies.
- **Leukocytes:** Several types of leukocytes (also known as White Blood Cells) are critical to the process of neutralizing invading substance. Neutrophils, for example, are small and agile and are able to first arrive at the scene of the crime to ingest small microbes. However, large substances such as Macrophages as required to tackle a large number of microbes.

There are a few more, but the gist still remains the same. When your body starts to suffer from an uncontrolled inflammation attack, the action of these and similar substances tend to go out of control, which results in extremely uncomfortable situations.

The harmful side effects of Inflammation

Uncontrolled inflammation results in diseases that are known as "Autoimmune diseases. While there is a large number of them out there, some of the more prominent are as follows:

- **Type 1 Diabetes:** Type 1 Diabetes will cause the immune system to attack and destroy insulin-producing cells in your pancreas that will completely disrupt the regulation of sugar levels in your body.
- **Rheumatoid Arthritis:** RA causes the immune system to attack certain joints that results in great discomfort and pain.
- **Psoriatic Arthritis:** This causes the skin cell to multiply rapidly, which results in red and scaly patches called plaques on the skin.
- **Multiple Sclerosis:** MS tends to damage the protective coating that surrounds nerve cells (known as myelin sheath) and affects the transmission of a neural message between the brain and body. This often leads to weakness, balance issues, etc.
- **Inflammatory Bowel Syndromes:** This disease will cause irritation of the intestinal lining.
- **Graves' Disease:** This disease attacks the thyroid gland in your neck and causes it to produce too much hormone, which results in a severe imbalance.
- **Cancer:** Cancerous tumors tend to secrete substances that attract cytokines and free-radicals that further cause inflammation and helps the tumors to survive. So, if you are already suffering from Anti-Inflammation, it will just make the condition of the Cancer much worse and help to grow and spread.
- **Alzheimer:** The brain does not have any pain receptors, but that doesn't mean that it won't be able to feel the effects of inflammation. Researchers have recently discovered that people a high level of Omega-6 fatty acids tend to have

a greater chance of suffering from Alzheimer's disease, which simply put is a disease and hampers your memory and makes you keep forgetting things from time to time.

Just to name a few.

Different symptoms of Inflammation

While there are different types of diseases that are caused by Inflammation, the early symptoms of them are very much similar. These include:

- Fatigue
- Muscle ache
- Low-grade fever
- Redness and swelling
- Numbness in your feet and hand
- Loss of hair
- Skin rash

These are often accompanied by the symptoms that are specific to any disease that the patient might be suffering from. So, for example, if you are suffering from Type-1 Diabetes, then asides from the above-mentioned problems, you are likely to experience extreme thirst, weight loss, etc.

So, as you can see, Inflammation is actually pretty serious and you should take it very seriously.

And if by any chance you face symptoms of inflammations, then fasting will greatly help you to deal with it.

Now that we are done with the basics, let's have a look the recipes!

Chapter 5

Breakfast Recipes

Eggs in A Hole

Serving: 2

Prep Time: 10 minutes

Cook Time: 10 minutes

Ingredients

- 2 and ½ slices whole wheat bread
- Olive oil spray
- Fresh ground pepper
- Hot sauce to taste
- Salt to taste
- 2 and ½ ounces avocado flesh, mashed
- 2 large eggs

Directions

1. Take your bread slices and make a hole in the middle using a cookie cutter

2. Season avocado mash with salt and pepper

3. Take a skillet and place it over medium-low heat, grease with cooking spray

4. Place bread slices and a cut portion in the skillet

5. Break the egg into the hole of the bread, cook until the egg properly settles down, season with more salt and pepper

6. Flip and cook the other side

7. Once done, transfer to a plate

8. Top the egg with avocado mash, hot sauce and crumble bread (made from the cut piece)

9. Enjoy!

Nutrition Values (Per Serving)

- Calories: 229
- Fat: 23g
- Carbohydrates: 10g
- Protein: 12g

Tomato and Egg Scramble

Serving: 2

Prep Time: 10 minutes

Cook Time: 5 minutes

Smart Points: 4

Ingredients

- 8 whole eggs
- ½ cup fresh basil, chopped
- 2 tablespoons olive oil
- ½ teaspoon red pepper flakes, crushed
- 1 cup grape tomatoes, chopped
- Salt and pepper to taste

Directions

1. Take a bowl and whisk in eggs, salt, pepper, red pepper flakes and mix well
2. Add tomatoes, basil, and mix
3. Take a skillet and place it over medium-high heat
4. Add egg mixture and cook for 5 minutes and cooked and scrambled
5. Enjoy!

Nutrition Values (Per Serving)

- Calories: 130
- Fat: 10g
- Carbohydrates: 8g
- Protein: 1.8g

Hearty Pancakes

Serving: 4

Prep Time: 10 minutes

Cook Time: 5 minutes

Ingredients

- 1 teaspoon salt
- ½ cup low-fat milk
- 1 cup all-purpose flour
- 1 teaspoon vanilla
- 4 beaten eggs
- 1 teaspoon baking soda
- 2 cups non-fat Greek yogurt

Directions

1. Add Greek yogurt to your bowl and mix in the dry ingredients in another bowl

2. Stir the mixture into your yogurt and make sure everything is mixed well

3. Stir in eggs, milk, vanilla and stir well

4. Stir the mixture into the yogurt batter and add more flour to thicken it up

5. Take a skillet and place it over medium heat, add pancake batter and cook until bubbles appear

6. Flip and cook the other side

7. Repeat with remaining batter and enjoy!

Nutrition Values (Per Serving)

- Calorie: 212
- Fat: 2g
- Carbohydrates: 28g
- Protein: 2g

Pineapple Oatmeal

Serving: 5

Prep Time: 10 minutes

Cook Time: 4-8 hours

Ingredients

- 1 cup steel-cut oats
- 4 cups unsweetened almond milk
- 2 medium apples, slashed
- 1 teaspoon coconut oil
- 1 teaspoon cinnamon
- ¼ teaspoon nutmeg
- 2 tablespoons maple syrup
- A drizzle of lemon juice

Directions

1. Add listed ingredients to a cooking pan and mix well

2. Cook on very low flame for 8 hours/ or on high flame for 4 hours

3. Gently stir

4. Add toppings your desired toppings

5. Serve and enjoy!

6. Store in the fridge for later use, make sure to add a splash of almond milk after re-heating for added flavor

Nutrition Values (Per Serving)

- Calories: 180
- Fat: 5g
- Carbohydrates: 31g
- Protein: 5g

Delicious Pumpkin Pie Oatmeal

Serving: 2

Prep Time: 10 minutes

Cook Time: 10 minutes

Ingredients

- ½ cup canned pumpkin
- Mashed banana as needed
- ¾ cup unsweetened almond milk
- ½ teaspoon pumpkin pie spice
- 1 cup oats
- 2 teaspoons maple syrup

Directions

1. Mash banana using fork and mix in the remaining ingredients (except oats) and mix well

2. Add oats and finely stir

3. Transfer mixture to a pot and let the oats cook until it has absorbed the liquid and are tender

4. Serve and enjoy!

Nutrition Values (Per Serving)

- Calories: 264
- Fat: 4g
- Carbohydrates: 52g
- Protein: 7g

Egg Muffins

Serving: 6

Prep Time: 10 minutes

Cook Time: 30 minutes

Ingredients

- ½ teaspoon sage
- ½ teaspoon pepper
- ¼ teaspoon red pepper flakes
- ½ pound ground turkey
- 1 bell pepper, diced
- 12 whole eggs
- ¼ teaspoon salt
- ¼ teaspoon Marjoram

Directions

1. Preheat your oven to 350 degrees F
2. Grease a cupcake tin with non-stick spray
3. Take a skillet and place it over medium heat, add turkey and cook
4. Beat in eggs with seasoning, stir in bell pepper and cooked turkey to the egg mixture
5. Divide egg mixture between muffin tins and bake for 30 minutes
6. Once the eggs are set, enjoy!

Nutrition Values (Per Serving)

- Calories: 172
- Fat: 10g
- Carbohydrates: 2g
- Protein: 16g

Chapter 6

Beef and Pork Recipes

Spicy Meatballs

Serving: 4

Prep Time: 10 minutes

Cook Time: 25 minutes + 2-4 hours

Ingredients

- 2 whole eggs
- 2 pounds organic beef, ground
- 4-5 tablespoons fruit-sweetened grape jelly
- 1/2 teaspoon pepper, ground
- ½ teaspoon Spanish paprika
- ¼ teaspoon chili powder
- 1 teaspoon ground garlic salt
- ¼ cup tapioca flour

Directions

1. Preheat your oven to 350 degrees F
2. Add beef, pepper, eggs, garlic, salt, tapioca starch in a bowl
3. Mix well and make balls
4. Transfer to a baking sheet
5. Bake for 25 minutes
6. Transfer to a pot and add chili sauce, paprika, grape jelly, and chili powder
7. Cook on very flame for 2-4 hours (use a crockpot if possible)
8. Enjoy!

Nutrition Values (Per Serving)

- Calories: 288
- Fat: 4.6g
- Carbohydrates: 34g
- Protein: 2g

Mongolian Beef

Serving: 4

Prep Time: 10 minutes

Cook Time: 20

Ingredients

- 2 teaspoons Asian garlic chili paste
- 2 teaspoons vegetable oil
- 1 tablespoon rice vinegar
- 1 pound sirloin beef, lean and cubed
- 16 green onions, chopped
- 1 tablespoon ginger minced
- 2 tablespoons low soy sauce
- 1 garlic clove, minced
- 1 teaspoon cornstarch
- 1 tablespoon hoisin sauce

Directions

1. Take a bowl and stir in soy sauce, cornstarch, hoisin sauce, rice vinegar, chili paste
2. Add ginger, garlic, beef to a heated skillet and Saute for 3 minutes until the beef is nice and golden
3. Mix in sauce, green onions and cook for a few minutes
4. Enjoy!

Nutrition Values (Per Serving)

- Calorie: 231
- Fat: 7g
- Carbohydrates: 10g
- Protein: 27g

Western Pork Chops

Serving: 4

Prep Time: 10 minutes

Cook Time: 15 minutes

Ingredients

- Cooking spray as needed
- 4-ounce pork loin chop, boneless and fat rimmed
- 1/3 cup of salsa
- 2 tablespoon of fresh lime juice
- A ¼ cup of fresh cilantro, chopped

Directions

1. Take a large-sized non-stick skillet and spray it with cooking spray
2. Heat it up until hot over high heat
3. Press the chops with your palm to flatten them slightly
4. Add them to the skillet and cook on 1 minute for each side until they are nicely browned
5. Lower down the heat to medium-low
6. Combine the salsa and lime juice
7. Pour the mix over the chops
8. Simmer uncovered for about 8 minutes until the chops are perfectly done
9. If needed, sprinkle some cilantro on top
10. Serve!

Nutrition Values (Per Serving)

- Calorie: 184
- Fat: 4g
- Carbohydrates: 4g
- Protein: 0.5g

Smothered Pork Chops

Serving: 4

Prep Time: 10 minutes

Cook Time: 30 minutes

Ingredients

- 4 pork chops, bone-in
- 2 tablespoon of olive oil
- A ¼ cup of vegetable broth
- ½ a pound of Yukon gold potatoes, peeled and chopped
- 1 large onion, sliced
- 2 garlic cloves, minced
- 2 teaspoon of rubbed sage
- 1 teaspoon of thyme, ground
- Salt and pepper as needed

Directions

1. Preheat your oven to 350 degrees Fahrenheit
2. Take a large-sized skillet and place it over medium heat
3. Add a tablespoon of oil and allow the oil to heat up
4. Add pork chops and cook them for 4-5 minutes per side until browned
5. Transfer chops to a baking dish
6. Pour broth over the chops
7. Add remaining oil to the pan and Saute potatoes, onion, garlic for 3-4 minutes
8. Take a large bowl and add potatoes, garlic, onion, thyme, sage, pepper, and salt
9. Transfer this mixture to the baking dish (with pork)
10. Bake for 20-30 minutes
11. Serve and enjoy!

Nutrition Values (Per Serving)

- Calorie: 261
- Fat: 10g
- Carbohydrates: 1.3g
- Protein: 2g

Spicy Pork Chops

Serving: 4

Prep Time: 4 hours 10 minutes

Cook Time: 15 minutes

Ingredients

- ¼ cup lime juice
- 4 pork rib chops
- 1 tablespoon coconut oil, melted
- 2 garlic cloves, peeled and minced
- 1 tablespoon chili powder
- 1 teaspoon ground cinnamon
- 2 teaspoons cumin
- Salt and pepper to taste
- ½ teaspoon hot pepper sauce
- Mango, sliced

How To

1. Take a bowl and mix in lime juice, oil, garlic, cumin, cinnamon, chili powder, salt, pepper, hot pepper sauce
2. Whisk well
3. Add pork chops and toss
4. Keep it on the side and let it refrigerate for 4 hours
5. Pre-heat your grill to medium and transfer pork chops to a pre-heated grill
6. Grill for 7 minutes, flip and cook for 7 minutes more
7. Divide between serving platters and serve with mango slices
8. Enjoy!

Nutrition (Per Serving)

- Calories: 200
- Fat: 8g
- Carbohydrates: 3g
- Protein: 26g

Mediterranean Pork

Serving: 4

Prep Time: 10 minutes

Cook Time: 35 minutes

Ingredients

- 4 pork chops, bone-in
- Salt and pepper to taste
- 1 teaspoon dried rosemary
- 3 garlic cloves, peeled and minced

How To

1. Season pork chops with salt and pepper
2. Place in roasting pan
3. Add rosemary, garlic in a pan
4. Preheat your oven to 425 degrees F
5. Bake for 10 minutes
6. Lower heat to 350 degrees F
7. Roast for 25 minutes more
8. Slice pork and divide on plates
9. Drizzle pan juice all over
10. Serve and enjoy!

Nutrition (Per Serving)

- Calories: 165
- Fat: 2g
- Carbohydrates: 2g
- Protein: 26g

Paprika Lamb Chops

Serving: 4

Prep Time: 10 minutes

Cook Time: 15 minutes

Ingredients

- 2 lamb racks, cut into chops
- Salt and pepper to taste
- 3 tablespoons paprika
- ¾ cup cumin powder
- 1 teaspoon chili powder

How To

1. Take a bowl and add paprika, cumin, chili, salt, pepper, and stir
2. Add lamb chops and rub the mixture
3. Heat grill over medium-temperature and add lamb chops, cook for 5 minutes
4. Flip and cook for 5 minutes more, flip again
5. Cook for 2 minutes, flip and cook for 2 minutes more
6. Serve and enjoy!

Nutrition (Per Serving)

- Calories: 200
- Fat: 5g
- Carbohydrates: 4g
- Protein: 8g

Chapter 6

Poultry Recipes

Delicious Turkey Wrap

Serving: 6

Prep Time: 10 minutes

Cook Time: 10 minutes

<u>Ingredients</u>

- 1 and a ¼ pounds of ground turkey, lean
- 4 green onions, minced
- 1 tablespoon of olive oil
- 1 garlic clove, minced
- 2 teaspoon of chili paste
- 8-ounce water chestnut, diced
- 3 tablespoon of hoisin sauce
- 2 tablespoon of coconut aminos
- 1 tablespoon of rice vinegar
- 12 butter lettuce leaves
- 1/8 teaspoon of salt

<u>How To</u>

1. Take a pan and place it over medium heat, add turkey and garlic to the pan
2. Heat for 6 minutes until cooked
3. Take a bowl and transfer turkey to the bowl
4. Add onions and water chestnuts
5. Stir in hoisin sauce, coconut aminos, vinegar, and chili paste
6. Toss well and transfer the mix to lettuce leaves
7. Serve and enjoy!

<u>Nutrition (Per Serving)</u>

- Calories: 162
- Fat: 4g
- Net Carbohydrates: 7g
- Protein: 23g

Bacon and Chicken Garlic Wrap

Serving: 4

Prep Time: 15 minutes

Cook Time: 10 minutes

Ingredients

- 1 chicken fillet, cut into small cubes
- 8-9 thin slices bacon, cut to fit cubes
- 6 garlic cloves, minced

How To

1. Preheat your oven to 400 degrees F
2. Line a baking tray with aluminum foil
3. Add minced garlic to a bowl and rub each chicken piece with it
4. Wrap bacon piece around each garlic chicken bite
5. Secure with toothpick
6. Transfer bites to the baking sheet, keeping a little bit of space between them
7. Bake for about 15-20 minutes until crispy
8. Serve and enjoy!

Nutrition (Per Serving)

- Calories: 260
- Fat: 19g
- Carbohydrates: 5g
- Protein: 22g

Blackened Chicken

Serving: 4

Prep Time: 10 minutes

Cook Time: 10 minutes

Ingredients

- ½ teaspoon paprika
- 1/8 teaspoon salt
- ¼ teaspoon cayenne pepper
- ¼ teaspoon ground cumin
- ¼ teaspoon dried thyme
- 1/8 teaspoon ground white pepper
- 1/8 teaspoon onion powder
- 2 chicken breasts, boneless and skinless

How To

1. Preheat your oven to 350 degrees Fahrenheit

2. Grease baking sheet

3. Take a cast-iron skillet and place it over high heat

4. Add oil and heat it up for 5 minutes until smoking hot

5. Take a small bowl and mix salt, paprika, cumin, white pepper, cayenne, thyme, onion powder

6. Oil the chicken breast on both sides and coat the breast with the spice mix

7. Transfer to your hot pan and cook for 1 minute per side

8. Transfer to your prepared baking sheet and bake for 5 minutes

9. Serve and enjoy!

Nutrition (Per Serving)

- Calories: 136
- Fat: 3g
- Carbohydrates: 1g
- Protein: 24g

Chicken Garlic Platter

Serving: 6

Prep Time: 5 minutes

Cook Time: 10 minutes

Ingredients

- 3 large chicken breast
- 10-ounces spinach, frozen and drained
- 3-ounce mozzarella cheese, part-skim
- ½ a cup of roasted red peppers, cut in long strips
- 1 teaspoon of olive oil
- 2 garlic cloves, minced
- Salt and pepper as needed

How To

1. Preheat your oven to 400 degrees Fahrenheit
2. Slice 3 chicken breast lengthwise
3. Take a non-stick pan and grease with cooking spray
4. Bake for 2-3 minutes each side
5. Take another skillet and cook spinach and garlic in oil for 3 minutes
6. Place chicken on an oven pan and top with spinach, roasted peppers, and mozzarella
7. Bake until the cheese melted
8. Enjoy!

Nutrition (Per Serving)

- Calories: 195
- Fat: 7g
- Net Carbohydrates: 3g
- Protein: 30g

Clean Parsley and Chicken Breast

Serving: 4

Prep Time: 10 minutes

Cook Time: 40 minutes

Ingredients

- 1 tablespoon dry parsley
- 1 tablespoon dry basil
- 4 chicken breast halves, boneless and skinless
- ½ teaspoon salt
- ½ teaspoon red pepper flakes, crushed
- 2 tomatoes, sliced

How To

1. Preheat your oven to 350 degrees F
2. Take a 9x13 inch baking dish and grease it up with cooking spray
3. Sprinkle 1 tablespoon of parsley, 1 teaspoon of basil and spread the mixture over your baking dish
4. Arrange the chicken breast halves over the dish and sprinkle garlic slices on top
5. Take a small bowl and add 1 teaspoon parsley, 1 teaspoon of basil, salt, basil, red pepper and mix well. Pour the mixture over the chicken breast
6. Top with tomato slices and cover, bake for 25 minutes
7. Remove the cover and bake for 15 minutes more
8. Serve and enjoy!

Nutrition (Per Serving)

- Calories: 150
- Fat: 4g
- Carbohydrates: 4g
- Protein: 25g

Balsamic Chicken

Serving: 6

Prep Time: 10 minutes

Cook Time: 25 minutes

Ingredients

- 6 chicken breast halves, skinless and boneless
- 1 teaspoon garlic salt
- Ground black pepper
- 2 tablespoons olive oil
- 1 onion, thinly sliced
- 14 and ½ ounces tomatoes, diced
- ½ cup balsamic vinegar
- 1 teaspoon dried basil
- 1 teaspoon dried oregano
- 1 teaspoon dried rosemary
- ½ teaspoon dried thyme

How To

1. Season both sides of your chicken breasts thoroughly with pepper and garlic salt

2. Take a skillet and place it over medium heat

3. Add some oil and cook your seasoned chicken for 3-4 minutes per side until the breasts are nicely browned

4. Add some onion and cook for another 3-4 minutes until the onions are browned

5. Pour the diced up tomatoes and balsamic vinegar over your chicken and season with some rosemary, basil, thyme, and rosemary

6. Simmer the chicken for about 15 minutes until they are no longer pink

7. Take an instant-read thermometer and check if the internal temperature gives a reading of 165 degrees Fahrenheit

8. If yes, then you are good to go!

Nutrition (Per Serving)

- Calories: 196
- Fat: 7g
- Carbohydrates: 7g
- Protein: 23g

Chapter 7

Snacks and Appetizers Recipes

Cheese Mug

Serving: 1

Prep Time: 4 minutes

Cook Time: 1-2 minutes

Ingredients

- 2 ounces roast beef slices
- 1 and ½ tablespoons green chilies, diced
- 1 and ½ ounces pepper jack cheese, shredded
- 1 tablespoon sour cream

How To

1. Layer roast beef on the bottom of your mug, making sure to break it down into small pieces

2. Add half a tablespoon of sour cream, add half tablespoon green Chile and half an ounce of pepper jack cheese

3. Keep layering until all ingredients are used

4. Microwave for 2 minutes

5. Server warm and enjoy!

Nutrition (Per Serving)

- Calories: 268
- Fat: 16g
- Carbohydrates: 4g
- Protein: 22g

Lemon Broccoli

Serving: 4

Prep Time: 10 minutes

Cook Time: 15 minutes

Ingredients

- 2 heads broccoli, separated into florets
- 2 teaspoons extra virgin olive oil
- 1 teaspoon salt
- ½ teaspoon pepper
- 1 garlic clove, minced
- ½ teaspoon lemon juice

How To

1. Pre-heat your oven to a temperature of 400 degrees F
2. Take a large-sized bowl and add broccoli florets with some extra virgin olive oil, pepper, sea salt and garlic
3. Spread the broccoli out in a single even layer on a fine baking sheet
4. Bake in your pre-heated oven for about 15-20 minutes until the florets are soft enough so that they can be pierced with a fork
5. Squeeze lemon juice over them generously before serving
6. Enjoy!

Nutrition (Per Serving)

- Calories: 49
- Fat: 2g
- Carbohydrates: 4g
- Protein: 3g

Stuffed Mushrooms

Serving: 4

Prep Time: 10 minutes

Cook Time: 15 minutes

Ingredients

- 4 Portobello mushroom
- 1 cup crumbled blue cheese
- 2 teaspoons extra virgin olive oil
- Salt, to taste
- Fresh thyme

How To

1. Preheat your oven to 350 degrees Fahrenheit
2. Put out the stems from the mushrooms
3. Chop them into small pieces
4. Take a bowl and mix stem pieces with thyme, salt, and blue cheese and mix well
5. Fill up mushroom with the prepared cheese
6. Top them with some oil
7. Take a baking sheet and place the mushrooms
8. Bake for 15 minutes to 20 minutes
9. Serve warm and enjoy!

Nutrition (Per Serving)

- Calories: 124
- Fat: 22.4g
- Carbohydrates: 5.4g
- Protein: 1.2g

Garlic Bread Stick

Serving: 8 breadsticks

Prep Time: 15 minutes

Cook Time: 15 minutes

Ingredients

- ¼ cup butter softened
- 1 teaspoon garlic powder
- 2 cups almond flour
- ½ tablespoon baking powder
- 1 tablespoon Psyllium husk powder
- ¼ teaspoon salt
- 3 tablespoons butter, melted
- 1 egg
- ¼ cup boiling water

How To

1. Preheat your oven to 400 degrees F
2. Line baking sheet with parchment paper and keep it on the side
3. Beat butter with garlic powder and keep it on the side
4. Add almond flour, baking powder, husk, salt in a bowl and mix in butter and egg, mix well
5. Pour boiling water in the mix and stir until you have a nice dough
6. Divide the dough into 8 balls and roll into breadsticks
7. Place on a baking sheet and bake for 15 minutes
8. Brush each stick with garlic butter and bake for 5 minutes more
9. Serve and enjoy!

Nutrition (Per Serving)

- Calories: 259
- Fat: 24g
- Carbohydrates: 5g
- Protein: 7g

Camembert Mushrooms

Serving: 4

Prep Time: 5 minutes

Cook Time: 13 minutes

Ingredients

- 2 tablespoons butter
- 4 ounces Camembert cheese, diced
- 2 teaspoons garlic, minced
- 1 pound button mushrooms, halved
- Black pepper to taste

How To

1. Place a skillet over medium-high heat

2. Add butter and let it melt

3. Once the butter has melted, add garlic and Saute until translucent, should take 3 minutes

4. Add mushrooms and cook for 10 minutes

5. Season with pepper and serve

6. Enjoy!

Nutrition (Per Serving)

- Calories: 161
- Fat: 13g
- Carbohydrates: 3g
- Protein: 9g

Eggplant Fries

Serving: 8

Prep Time: 10 minutes

Cook Time: 15 minutes

Ingredients

- 2 eggs
- 2 cups almond flour
- 2 tablespoons coconut oil, spray
- 2 eggplant, peeled and cut thinly
- Salt and pepper

How To

1. Preheat your oven to 400 degrees Fahrenheit
2. Take a bowl and mix with salt and black pepper in it
3. Take another bowl and beat eggs until frothy
4. Dip the eggplant pieces into eggs
5. Then coat them with flour mixture
6. Add another layer of flour and egg
7. Then, take a baking sheet and grease with coconut oil on top
8. Bake for about 15 minutes
9. Serve and enjoy!

Nutrition (Per Serving)

- Calories: 212
- Fat: 15.8g
- Carbohydrates: 12.1g
- Protein: 8.6g

Parmesan Crisps

Serving: 8

Prep Time: 5 minutes

Cook Time: 25 minutes

Ingredients

- 1 teaspoon butter
- 8 ounces parmesan cheese, full fat and shredded

How To

1. Preheat your oven to 400 degrees F
2. Put parchment paper on a baking sheet and grease with butter
3. Spoon parmesan into 8 mounds, spreading them apart evenly
4. Flatten them
5. Bake for 5 minutes until browned
6. Let them cool
7. Serve and enjoy!

Nutrition (Per Serving)

- Calories: 133
- Fat: 11g
- Carbohydrates: 1g
- Protein: 11g

Roasted Broccoli

Serving: 4

Prep Time: 5 minutes

Cook Time: 20 minutes

Ingredients

- 4 cups broccoli florets
- 1 tablespoon olive oil
- Salt and pepper to taste

How To

1. Preheat your oven to 400 degrees F
2. Add broccoli in a zip bag alongside oil and shake until coated
3. Add seasoning and shake again
4. Spread broccoli out on the baking sheet, bake for 20 minutes
5. Let it cool and serve
6. Enjoy!

Nutrition (Per Serving)

- Calories: 62
- Fat: 4g
- Carbohydrates: 4g
- Protein: 4g

Chapter 8

Fish and Seafood Recipes

Tuna Croquet

Serving: 4

Prep Time: 4 minutes

Cook Time: 9 minutes

Ingredients

- 1 can tuna, drained
- 1 whole large egg
- 8 tablespoons parmesan cheese, grated
- 2 tablespoons flax meal
- Salt and pepper to taste
- 1 tablespoons onion, minced

How To

1. Add all of the ingredients to a blender (except flax meal) and pulse the mixture into a crunchy texture
2. Form patties using the mixture
3. Dip both sides of the patties in flax meals and fry them in hot oil until both sides are browned well

Nutrition (Per Serving)

- Calories: 105
- Fat: 5g
- Carbohydrates: 2g
- Protein: 14g

Tuna Bites

Serving: 2

Prep Time: 10 minutes

Cook Time: 10 minutes

Ingredients

- 10 ounces of Canned Tuna, drained
- ¼ cup Keto-Friendly mayonnaise
- 1 medium avocado, cubed
- ¼ cup parmesan cheese
- 1/3 cup almond flour
- ½ teaspoon garlic powder
- ¼ teaspoon onion powder
- Salt and pepper as needed
- ½ cup of coconut oil

How To

1. Take a mixing bowl and add the listed ingredients except for coconut oil and avocado
2. Take the cubed avocado and carefully fold them in the tuna mix
3. Mix well and turn the mixture into balls
4. Roll the balls into almond flour
5. Take a pan over medium heat and add coconut oil
6. Allow the oil to heat up
7. Add tuna balls and cook them well until you have a brown texture
8. Serve and enjoy!

Nutrition (Per Serving)

- Calories: 134
- Fat: 11g
- Carbohydrates: 2g
- Protein: 7g

Simple Baked Shrimp with Béchamel Sauce

Serving: 4

Prep Time: 10 minutes

Cook Time: 5-7 minutes

Ingredients

- 6-7 ounces shrimp
- 1-ounces mozzarella
- 4 ounces béchamel sauce (recipe provided)
- 1 tablespoons ghee

How To

1. Cut boiled shrimp and transfer them to a baking dish
2. Pour sauce on top
3. Bake for 5-7 minutes
4. Serve and enjoy!

Nutrition (Per Serving)

- Calories: 150
- Fat: 10g
- Carbohydrates: 2g
- Protein: 14g

Grilled Lime Shrimp

Serving: 8

Prep Time: 25 minutes

Cook Time: 5 minutes

Ingredients

- 1 pound medium shrimp, peeled and deveined
- 1 lime, juiced
- ½ cup olive oil
- 3 tablespoons Cajun seasoning

How To

1. Take a re-sealable zip bag and add lime juice, Cajun seasoning, olive oil
2. Add shrimp and shake it well, let it marinate for 20 minutes
3. Preheat your outdoor grill to medium heat
4. Lightly grease the grate
5. Remove shrimp from marinade and cook for 2 minutes per side
6. Serve and enjoy!

Nutrition (Per Serving)

- Calories: 188
- Fat: 3g
- Net Carbohydrates: 1.2g
- Protein: 13g

Mouthwatering Calamari

Serving: 4

Prep Time: 10 minutes +1 hour marinating

Cook Time: 8 minutes

Ingredients

- 2 tablespoons extra virgin olive oil
- 1 teaspoon chili powder
- ½ teaspoon ground cumin
- Zest of 1 lime
- Juice of 1 lime
- Dash of sea salt
- 1 and ½ pounds squid, cleaned and split open, with tentacles cut into ½ inch rounds
- 2 tablespoons cilantro, chopped
- 2 tablespoons red bell pepper, minced

How To

1. Take a medium bowl and stir in olive oil, chili powder, cumin, lime zest, sea salt, lime juice, and pepper
2. Add squid and let it marinade and stir to coat, coat and let it refrigerate for 1 hour
3. Pre-heat your oven to broil
4. Arrange squid on a baking sheet, broil for 8 minutes turn once until tender
5. Garnish the broiled calamari with cilantro and red bell pepper
6. Serve and enjoy!

Nutrition (Per Serving)

- Calories: 159
- Fat: 13g
- Carbohydrates: 12g
- Protein: 3g

Glazed Salmon

Serving: 4

Prep Time: 45 minutes

Cook Time: 10 minutes

Ingredients

- 4 pieces salmon fillets, 5 ounces each
- 4 tablespoons coconut aminos
- 4 teaspoon olive oil
- 2 teaspoon ginger, minced
- 4 teaspoon garlic, minced
- 2 tablespoon sugar-free ketchup
- 4 tablespoons dry white wine
- 2 tablespoons red boat fish sauce

How To

1. Take a bowl and mix in coconut aminos, garlic, ginger, fish sauce, and mix
2. Add salmon and let it marinate for 15-20 minutes
3. Take a skillet/pan and place it over medium heat
4. Add oil and let it heat up
5. Add salmon fillets and cook on HIGH for 3-4 minutes per side
6. Remove dish once crispy
7. Add sauce and wine
8. Simmer for 5 minutes on low heat
9. Return salmon to the glaze and flip until both sides are glazed
10. Serve and enjoy!

Nutrition (Per Serving)

- Calories: 200
- Fat: 24g
- Carbohydrates: 3g
- Protein: 35g

Chapter 9

Vegetarian Recipes

Zucchini and Onions in A Single Lovely Platter

Serving: 4

Prep Time: 15 minutes

Cook Time: 45 minutes

Ingredients

- 3 large zucchinis, julienned
- 1 cup cherry tomatoes, halved
- ½ cup basil
- 2 red onions, thinly sliced
- ¼ teaspoon salt
- 1 teaspoon cayenne pepper
- 2 tablespoons lemon juice

How To

1. Create zucchini Zoodles by using a vegetable peeler and shaving the zucchini with peeler lengthwise, until you get to the core and seeds
2. Turn zucchini and repeat until you have long strips
3. Discard seeds
4. Lay strips on cutting board and slice lengthwise to your desired thickness
5. Mix Zoodles in a bowl alongside onion, basil, tomatoes, and toss
6. Sprinkle salt and cayenne pepper on top
7. Drizzle lemon juice
8. Serve and enjoy!

Nutrition (Per Serving)

- Calories: 156
- Fat: 8g
- Carbohydrates: 6g
- Protein: 7g

Collard Greens

Serving: 6

Prep Time: 10 minutes

Cook Time: 60 minutes

Ingredients

- 1 tablespoon olive oil
- 3 bacon, sliced
- 1 large onion, chopped
- 2 garlic cloves, minced
- 1 teaspoon salt
- 3 cups chicken broth
- 1 red pepper flake
- 1 pound fresh collard greens, cut into 2 inch pieces

How To

1. Take a large-sized pan and place it over medium-high heat
2. Add oil and allow the oil to heat it up
3. Add bacon and cook it until crispy and remove it, crumble the bacon and add the crumbled bacon to the pan
4. Add onion and keep cooking for 5 minutes
5. Add garlic and cook until a nice fragrant comes
6. Add collard greens and keep frying until wilt, add chicken broth and season with pepper, salt, and red pepper flakes
7. Lower down the heat and cover with a lid, simmer for 45 minutes
8. Enjoy!

Nutrition (Per Serving)

- Calories: 127
- Fat: 10g
- Carbohydrates: 8g
- Protein: 4g

Leeks Platter

Serving: 6

Prep Time: 10 minutes

Cook Time: 25 minutes

Ingredients

- 1 and ½ pound leeks, trimmed and chopped into 4-inch pieces
- 2 ounces butter
- 1 cup coconut cream
- 3 and ½ ounces cheddar cheese
- Salt and pepper to taste

How To

1. Preheat your oven to 400 degrees F
2. Take a skillet and place it over medium heat, add butter and let it heat up
3. Add leeks and Saute for 5 minutes
4. Spread leeks in a greased baking dish
5. Boil cream in a saucepan and lower heat to low
6. Stir in cheese, salt, and pepper
7. Pour sauce over leeks
8. Bake for 15-20 minutes and serve warm
9. Enjoy!

Nutrition (Per Serving)

- Calories: 204
- Fat: 15g
- Carbohydrates: 9g
- Protein: 7g

Broccoli and Cauliflower

Serving: 4

Prep Time: 10 minutes

Cook Time: 10 minutes

Ingredients

- 1 pound broccoli, chopped
- 2 ounces butter
- 8 ounces cauliflower, chopped
- 5 and 1/3 ounces shredded cheese
- Salt and pepper, to taste
- 4 teaspoons sour cream

How To

1. Take a large skillet and melt butter
2. Stir in all the vegetables
3. Sauté until it turns into golden brown over medium-high heat
4. Add all the remaining ingredients to the vegetable
5. Mix well
6. Serve warm and enjoy!

Nutrition (Per Serving)

- Calories: 244
- Fat: 20.5g
- Carbohydrates: 3.4g
- Protein: 12.2g

Zucchini BBQ

Serving: 1

Prep Time: 10 minutes

Cook Time: 1 hour

Ingredients

- Olive oil as needed
- 3 zucchinis
- ½ teaspoon black pepper
- ½ teaspoon mustard
- ½ teaspoon cumin
- 1 teaspoon paprika
- 1 teaspoon garlic powder
- 1 tablespoon of sea salt
- 1-2 stevia
- 1 tablespoon chili powder

How To

1. Preheat your oven to 300 degrees F

2. Take a small bowl and add cayenne, black pepper, salt, garlic, mustard, paprika, chili powder, and stevia

3. Mix well

4. Slice zucchini into 1/8 inch slices and mist them with olive oil

5. Sprinkle spice blend over zucchini and bake for 40 minutes

6. Remove and flip, mist with more olive oil and leftover spice

7. Bake for 20 minutes more

8. Serve!

Nutrition (Per Serving)

- Calories: 163
- Fat: 14g
- Carbohydrates: 3g
- Protein: 8g

Bok Choy Samba

Serving: 3

Prep Time: 5 minutes

Cook Time: 15 minutes

Ingredients

- 4 bok choy, sliced
- 1 onion, sliced
- ½ cup Parmesan cheese, grated
- 4 teaspoons coconut cream
- Salt and freshly ground black pepper, to taste

How To

1. Mix bok choy with black pepper and salt
2. Take a cooking pan, heat the oil and onion slice to sauté for 5 minutes
3. Then add cream and seasoned bok choy
4. Cook for 6 minutes
5. Stir in Parmesan cheese and cover the lid
6. Reduce the heat to low and cook for 3 minutes
7. Serve warm and enjoy!

Nutrition (Per Serving)

- Calories: 112
- Fat: 4.9g
- Carbohydrates: 1.9g
- Protein: 3g

Coconut and Cauliflower

Serving: 4

Prep Time: 20 minutes

Cook Time: 20 minutes

Ingredients

- 3 cups cauliflower, riced
- 2/3 cups full-fat coconut milk
- 1-2 teaspoons sriracha paste
- ¼- ½ teaspoon onion powder
- Salt as needed
- Fresh basil for garnish

How To

1. Take a pan and place it over medium-low heat
2. Add all of the ingredients and stir them until fully combined
3. Cook for about 5-10 minutes, making sure that the lid is on
4. Remove the lid and keep cooking until any excess liquid goes away
5. Once the rice is soft and creamy, enjoy!

Nutrition (Per Serving)

- Calories: 95
- Fat: 7g
- Carbohydrates: 4g
- Protein: 1g

Cauliflower Cake

Serving: 4

Prep Time: 10 minutes

Cook Time: 10 minutes

Ingredients

- 4 cups cauliflowers, cut into florets
- 1 cup cheddar cheese, grated
- 2 eggs, lightly beaten
- 1 teaspoon paprika
- 1 teaspoon chili powder
- Salt and pepper to taste
- ½ cup fresh parsley, chopped
- 1 tablespoon olive oil

How To

1. Add cauliflower, cheese, paprika, eggs, chili, salt, pepper and parsley into a large-sized bowl
2. Mix well
3. Drizzle olive oil into frying pan and place over medium-high heat
4. Shape cauliflower mixture into 12 even patties
5. Once the oil is hot, fry cakes until both sides are golden brown
6. Serve hot and enjoy!

Nutrition (Per Serving)

- Calories: 180
- Fat: 8g
- Carbohydrates: 6g
- Protein: 8g

Broccoli and Almond

Serving: 4

Prep Time: 5 minutes

Cook Time: 5 minutes

Ingredients

- 1 large head of broccoli, cut into florets
- ¼ cup slivered almonds
- 2 ounces feta cheese, crumbled
- 2 tablespoons olive oil
- Salt and pepper to taste
- Juice of a ½ lemon

How To

1. Steam broccoli in the microwave
2. Place cooked broccoli in a large bowl and add slivered almonds, feta cheese, salt, pepper, olive oil, and lemon juice
3. Stir well to combined
4. Serve and enjoy!

Nutrition (Per Serving)

- Calories: 190
- Fat: 13g
- Carbohydrates: 11g
- Protein: 9g

Asparagus Tart

Serving: 4

Prep Time: 10 minutes

Cook Time: 20 minutes

Ingredients

- 4 whole eggs
- 1 garlic clove, chopped
- Salt and pepper to taste
- 20 asparagus spears, woody ends removed
- ½ cup cheddar cheese, grated
- 2 tablespoons walnuts, chopped

How To

1. Preheat your oven to 375 degrees F
2. Grease a pie dish with butter
3. Place eggs, garlic, pepper and salt to a small bowl and beat using a fork
4. Pour egg mixture into your tray
5. Lay asparagus onto egg into one row
6. Sprinkle grated cheese over asparagus
7. Place in oven and cook for 12 minutes until cheese melts
8. Enjoy!

Nutrition (Per Serving)

- Calories: 160
- Fat: 10g
- Carbohydrates: 5g
- Protein: 12g

Garlic and Kale

Serving: 4

Prep Time: 5 minutes

Cook Time: 10 minutes

Ingredients

- 1 bunch kale
- 2 tablespoons olive oil
- 4 garlic cloves, minced

How To

1. Carefully tear the kale into bite-sized portions, making sure to remove the stem

2. Discard the stems

3. Take a large-sized pot and place it over medium heat

4. Add olive oil and let the oil heat up

5. Add garlic and stir for 2 minutes

6. Add kale and cook for 5-10 minutes

7. Serve!

Nutrition (Per Serving)

- Calories: 121
- Fat: 8g
- Carbohydrates: 5g
- Protein: 4g

Green Bean Roast

Serving: 4

Prep Time: 10 minutes

Cook Time: 20 minutes

Ingredients

- 1 whole egg
- 2 tablespoons olive oil
- Salt and pepper to taste
- 1 pound fresh green beans
- 5 and ½ tablespoons grated parmesan cheese

How To

1. Preheat your oven to 400 degrees F

2. Take a bowl and whisk in eggs with oil and spices

3. Add beans and mix well

4. Stir in parmesan cheese and pour the mix into baking pan (lined with parchment paper)

5. Bake for 15-20 minutes

6. Serve warm and enjoy!

Nutrition (Per Serving)

- Calories: 216
- Fat: 21g
- Carbohydrates: 7g
- Protein: 9g

Spiced Up Kale Chips

Serving: 4

Prep Time: 4 minutes

Cook Time: 29 minutes

Ingredients

- 2 large bunch kale, chopped into 4 pieces and stemmed
- 1 tablespoon olive oil
- 1/8 teaspoon salt
- 1 teaspoon chipotle powder
- ¼ cup parmesan cheese, shredded

How To

1. Wash kale thoroughly and dry, cut into 4-inch pieces
2. Preheat your oven to 250 degrees F
3. Take a baking sheet and line with parchment paper
4. Take a bowl and add kale, coat the kale with olive oil, chipotle, and cheese
5. Transfer the mix to a baking sheet
6. Bake for 19 minutes and check the crispiness
7. If you need more crispiness, bake for 9 minutes more
8. Serve and enjoy!

Nutrition (Per Serving)

- Calories: 37
- Fat: 3g
- Carbohydrates: 2g
- Protein: 1g

Conclusion

I would like to thank you again for purchasing the book and taking the time to go through the book as well.

I do hope that this book has been helpful and you found the information contained within the scriptures useful!

Keep in mind that you are not only limited to the recipes provided in this book! Just go ahead and keep on exploring until you find the best intermittent fasting plan that suits your needs!

Stay healthy and stay safe!

A short tale

Let me end this book on a high note, by sharing a tale of mine that inspired me to write this book.

As far as cheesy stories go, my one probably sits at somewhere around the top, but it is what it is.

So, up until a couple of years, I was considered as being your traditional "Fat" kid. I had a huge belly, with weight crossing the limits of healthy standards and swayed into the "Overweight" category.

And honestly speaking, at first, I accepted it. I was ready to look at myself as being the "Fat" successful kid on the block. I tried to stick that stature, but unfortunately, things didn't go well.

My Highschool and College results were pretty good, but the hurdles started to come after I entered the so-called "Real" life after completing my studies.

I was able to land a decent job at a game studio, but here's the thing. There's a limit up to which you can truly stay happy by just focusing on your career.

As my career kept going upward, my healthy, looks started to diminish more and more, and I just kept working and eating.

Then suddenly one day, depression hit me. And hit me hard!

I realized that no one really found me particularly attractive, my body was getting flooded with a number of different diseases and I was facing breathing problems while running, climbing up the stairs or even doing regular work.

The final nail to the coffin came when one day, I conjured up enough courage to ask my crush out, but she blatantly rejected me and told it to my face that I am completely out of her league and I was a fool to even dream of having her.

With a broken heart, I decided to turn my life around, and thus I started to look around the web for a diet program that would suit my needs.

While there was a huge load of them, the Intermittent Fasting programs piqued my interested the most since it seemed easy to follow, simple and versatile enough to allow me to easily incorporate it to my life.

So, took a stand and did it. At first, it was extremely difficult to fast for so long, I tried to follow the 16:8 program as well, but eventually I got the hang of it, and within a week or two, I started getting a result.

The first week saw a reduction of 0.5Kg. But the following week I was able to lose almost 1 and ½ kg of weight! That's huge.

I was inspired and I kept moving forward with the program.

Almost 6 months later, and by the blessing of God, I was able to look at myself with pride with the feeling that yes, I have finally accomplished my goal and achieved a nice and healthy physique.

And that's pretty much, that's the tale of how I was inspired to write this book.

If a lazy bum like me can change, I am pretty sure that each and every one of you has the potential to completely change your life for good following the intermittent Fasting program and a little bit of physical workout.

Regardless of what your inspiration might be, I bid you my warmest wishes and hope that you are able to succeed in your journey!